Jihène Marrakchi

Practical manual of videonystagmography

Jihène Marrakchi

Practical manual of videonystagmography

ScienciaScripts

Imprint

Any brand names and product names mentioned in this book are subject to trademark, brand or patent protection and are trademarks or registered trademarks of their respective holders. The use of brand names, product names, common names, trade names, product descriptions etc. even without a particular marking in this work is in no way to be construed to mean that such names may be regarded as unrestricted in respect of trademark and brand protection legislation and could thus be used by anyone.

Cover image: www.ingimage.com

This book is a translation from the original published under ISBN 978-613-8-41636-4.

Publisher:
Sciencia Scripts
is a trademark of
Dodo Books Indian Ocean Ltd. and OmniScriptum S.R.L publishing group

120 High Road, East Finchley, London, N2 9ED, United Kingdom
Str. Armeneasca 28/1, office 1, Chisinau MD-2012, Republic of Moldova, Europe
Printed at: see last page
ISBN: 978-620-6-02433-0

I thank

Mr BERNARD COHEN

For guiding me through my learning curve and helping me with this work

All teachers of the DIU "VESTIBULAR REEDUCATION

For their availability and the quality of their courses.

TABLE OF CONTENTS:

CHAPTER 1   2   **3**

CHAPTER 2   **14**

CHAPTER 3   **20**

CHAPTER 1
Introduction

Videonystagmography (VNG), developed since the 1990s in the daily practice of ENT specialists, has revolutionised vestibular functional investigations. It has far surpassed the old recording method using electrodes (electronystagmography).

VNG has made it possible to examine vestibular function by finely analysing eye movements, focusing in particular on the rapid, involuntary movement known as 'nystagmus'. Through the use of infrared cameras, the patient's eyes can be recorded instantly and analysed by software allowing the practitioner to make a rapid diagnosis. After an anatomical-physiological reminder of the vestibular system, we will detail in this work the principle, the steps of realization and the results of the VNG.

II-1: Anatomy of the vestibular system :

The vestibular system consists of two parts on each side: the peripheral vestibular apparatus and the vestibular pathways divided into peripheral and central contingents.

1 - Peripheral vestibular apparatus :

The inner ear, or labyrinth, is located within the petrous pyramid of the temporal bone. It comprises a set of bony cavities, or bony labyrinth, containing tubular structures forming the membranous labyrinth. Within the membranous labyrinth are the anterior cochlear sensory organ for hearing and   the sensory sensors vestibular systems specialised in detecting angular and linear accelerations of the head (Figure 1)

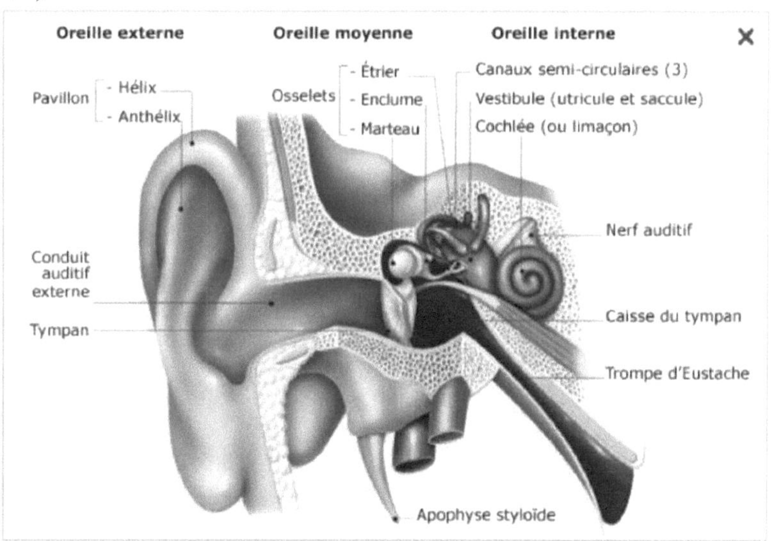

Figure 1: Overview of the ear with its three parts

1-1: The bony posterior labyrinth :

It comprises a central cavity (the vestibule) and the three semicircular canals: superior (anterior), horizontal (external) and posterior. Two canals from the bony labyrinth join the cerebral envelopes: the subarachnoid spaces for the limbic aqueduct and the dura mater for the vestibular aqueduct.

a/ the vestibule :

It is located between the tympanic cavity on the outside and the internal auditory canal on the inside. Its shape is irregular, globular as a whole. Its walls are hollowed out by the orifices of the semicircular canals, the oval window, the round window, and the outlet of the corkscrew and the aqueduct of the vestibule. They are also perforated by small openings, the sieve spots, which serve as passageways for the threads of the cochleovestibular nerve VIII (Figure 2). b/ the semicircular canals :

The semicircular canals (SCC) are three on each side and represent three arciform tubes forming an incomplete loop, each lying in a plane perpendicular to the other two. The right and left outer semicircular canals are located in the same plane and are said to be synergistic. The same is true for the right posterior and left superior semicircular canals, as well as the left posterior and right superior semicircular canals, which are in parallel planes. Each canal opens into the vestibule through its two ends, one of which is dilated and called ampullary. The non-ampullary ends of the superior and posterior canals join to form the common crus (Figure 3).

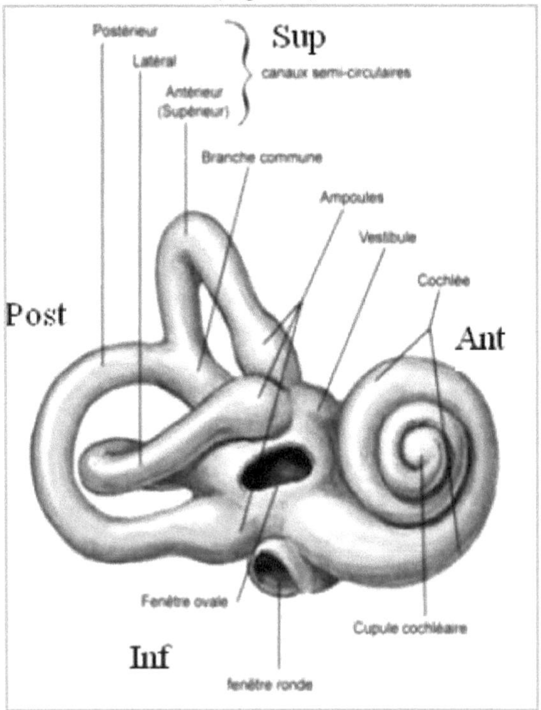

Figure 2: Anterolateral view of a bony labyrinth.

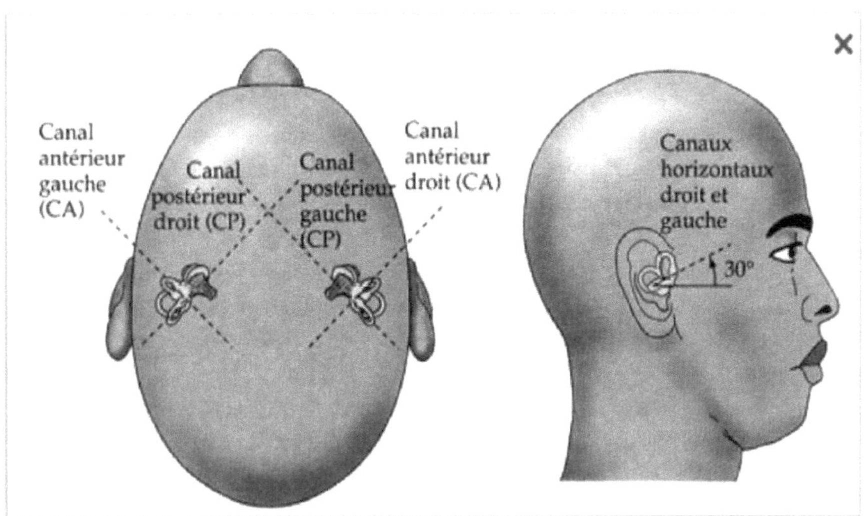

<u>Figure 3:</u> Representation of the six semicircular canals in space.

1-2: The posterior membranous labyrinth:

The membranous labyrinth is the set of cavities with a conjunctivo-epithelial wall that line the bony labyrinth. It contains the endolymphatic fluid and is surrounded by the perilymph.

It comprises the utricle and saccule which form the membranous vestibule and membranous CSCs and supports the neurosensory receptors.

a/ The membranous vestibule :

It consists of two vesicles contained in the bony vestibule: the utricle and the saccule.

<u>The utricle </u>is located in the elliptical fossa of the inner wall. It responds to the oval window and receives the outlet of the semicircular canals. The utricular macula is located on the anterior part of the floor of the utricle in a horizontal position.

<u>The saccule </u>is located in the hemispheric fossa of the bony vestibule. It communicates posteriorly with the sinus of the endolymphatic duct via the saccular duct, and anteriorly with the cochlear duct via the ductus réuniens.

The saccular macule is located on the vertical inner wall and is perpendicular to the utricular macule.

Each macule has a neurosensory epithelium on which the otolith membrane, containing the otoconia, rests.

Otoconia or otoliths are inert formations rich in calcium carbonate of high density. The base of the otolith layer is embedded in a gelatinous layer and the rest in a layer of mucopolysaccharides.

The maculcs are sensitive to linear acceleration and gravitational forces.

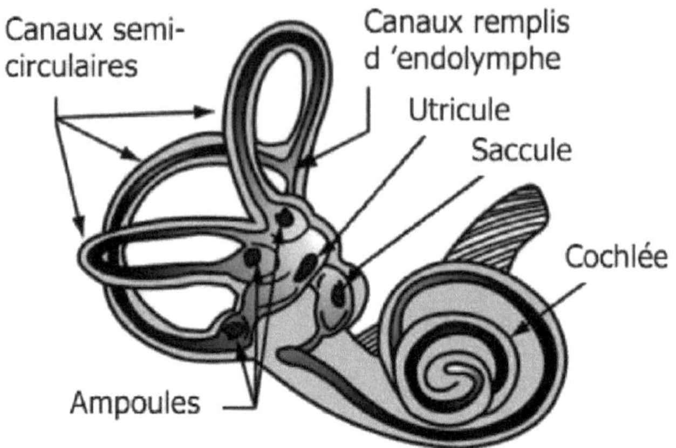

<u>Figure 4:</u> Diagram of the membranous vestibule.

b/The membranousCSCs :

At the level of each ampullary dilatation, there is a ridge which supports the sensory cells. It is surmounted by a cupula, partially obstructing the lumen of the canal. Each ridge is covered by a neuroepithelium comprising two types of cells: type I and type II cells. From here the afferent fibres of each ampullary nerve originate. The neurosensory receptors of the CSCs are sensitive to the angular acceleration of the head.

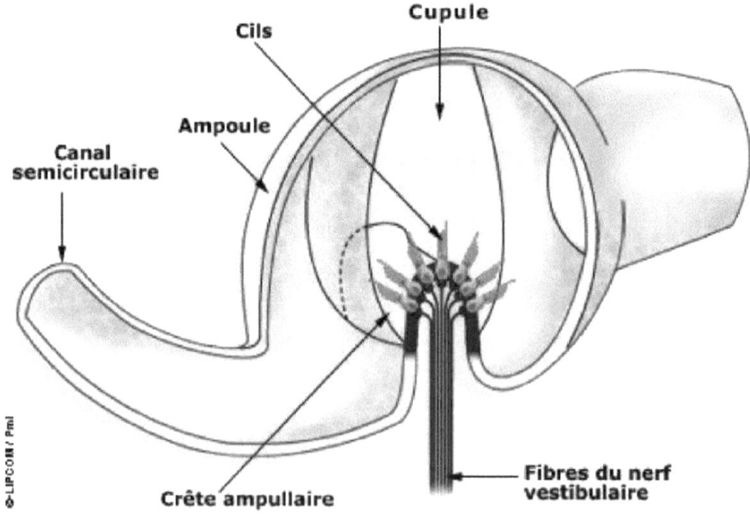

<u>Figure 5:</u> Representation of the ampullary ridge

2 -Vestibular pathways :

They consist of the vestibular nerve, vestibular nuclei and spinal, oculomotor and cortical afferents.

2-1: Vestibular nerve :

The vestibular nerve transmits information encoded by the vestibular hair cells to the vestibular nuclei. Its course is entirely intracranial.

At the entrance to the internal auditory canal, the vestibular nerve is subdivided into three branches: the superior vestibular nerve, the inferior vestibular or saccular nerve and the posterior ampullary nerve.

The superior vestibular ramus is composed of the union of the nerves of the vertical and horizontal semicircular canals and the utricular nerve.

The inferior vestibular ramus is composed of fibres from the saccular nerve.

At the bottom of the internal auditory canal, the nerve has a bulge which corresponds to the vestibular ganglion (or Scarpa's ganglion).

The cell bodies of the primary vestibular neurons are located at this level.

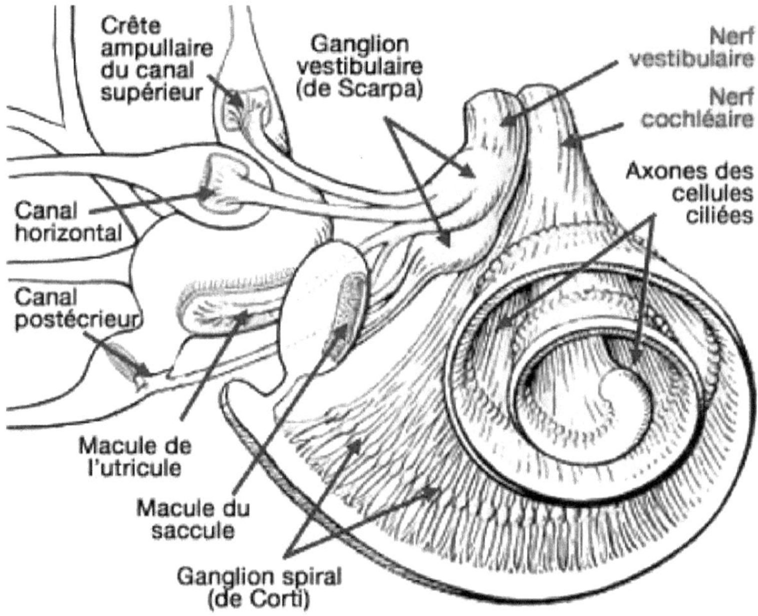

Figure 5: Representation of the vestibular nerve

As it passes through the internal auditory canal, the cochlear nerve and the facial nerve are located above and in front of it. This nerve bundle forms the acoustic-facial bundle. Finally, the vestibular nerve exits the canal through the porus located halfway up the posterior surface of the rock and reaches the pontocerebellar angle for a distance of 12 to 14 mm and then the encephalon.

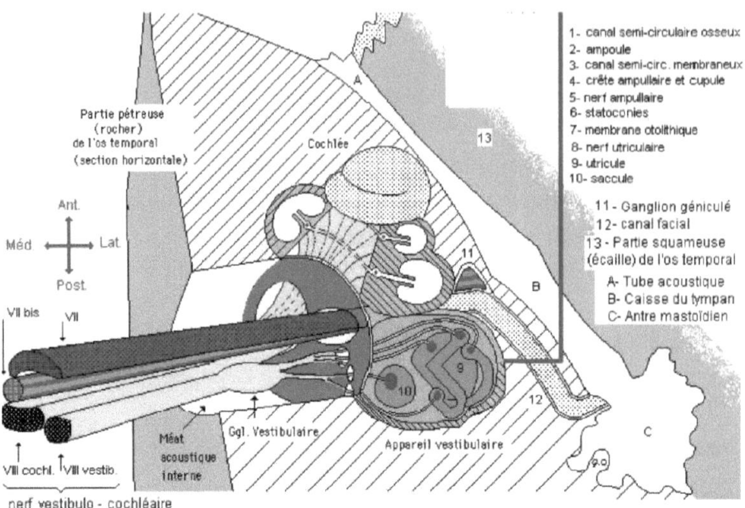

<u>Figure 6:</u> Representation of the origin and course of the vestibular nerve

Three <u>vestibular roots</u> are individualised:

* ascending root that leads to the medial and superior nuclei and the cerebellum.

* This is a descending root that leads to the inferior and medial nuclei through the lateral nucleus of Deiters.

*This is the only way to ensure that the brain is able to function properly and that it is able to function properly in the future.

2-2: The vestibular nuclei (Figures 8 and 9):

The vestibular nuclei are located on either side of the iveme ventricle, at the junction of the protuberance and the upper part of the bulb.

There are four main vestibular nuclei:

* the lateral vestibular nucleus (or nucleus of Deiters),

* the median core (Schwalbe),

* the lower (or descending) core

* the upper core.

These nuclei project via different bundles (lateral, medial and caudal vestibulospinal) to spinal motor neurons and via the medial longitudinal bundle (MLB) to oculomotor motor neurons. The superior vestibular nucleus is the only nucleus that does not send any direct projections to the spinal cord.

To this anatomical segmentation corresponds a functional segmentation.

<u>The canalicular afferents</u> project mainly to the superior vestibular nucleus, to the rostral and caudal parts of the inferior nucleus, to the medial nucleus and to a lesser extent to the medial part of the lateral nucleus.

<u>The utricular afferents</u> project to the ventral parts of the lateral nucleus, the rostral part

of the inferior nucleus and to a lesser extent to the medial nucleus.

The saccular afferents end mainly in the lateral and inferior nucleus.

In addition to these four main nuclei, there are also small cell groups (x, y, z, f, g and l), which also receive primary vestibular afferents, and which are mostly adjacent to the vestibular nuclei. The "y" group receives exclusively saccular projections.

The vestibular nuclei consist of vestibular neurons called secondary vestibular neurons and many other interneurons.

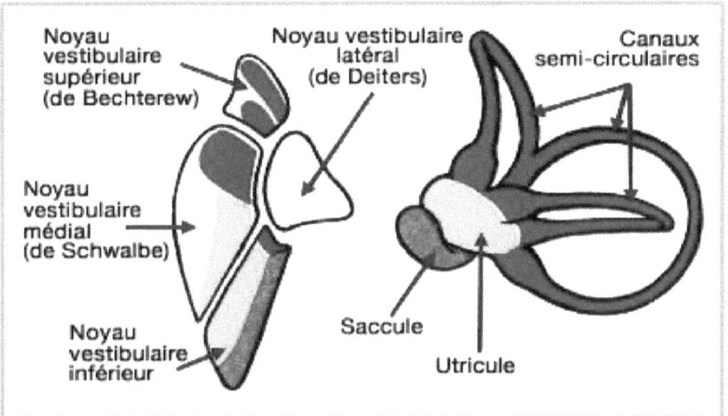

Figure 7: Representation of the afferents of the main vestibular nuclei

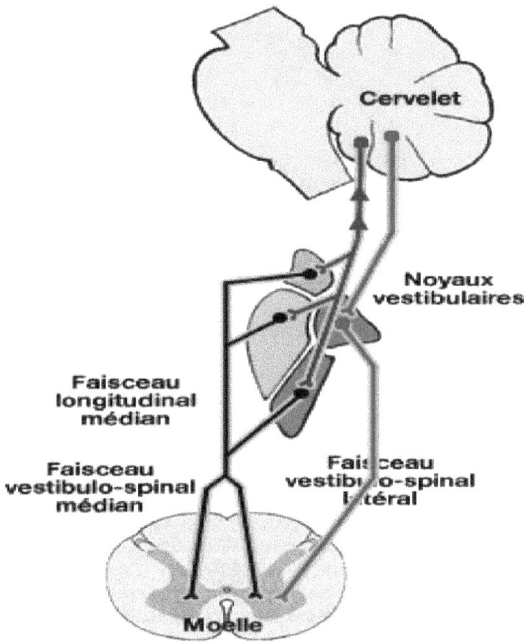

Figure 8: Representation of the projections of the main vestibular nuclei

2-3: Efferences :

a/ Vestibulo-oculomotor system:

It is a three-neuron reflex. It plays an important role in stabilising the image of the visual world during head movements. The vestibulo-ocular reflexes (VOR) induce slow compensatory movements of the eye in the same plane as the plane of head rotation but in the opposite direction. These slow phases, which have the same speed as the head movement, are followed by a rapid return phase (physiological ocular nystagmus), which allows the eye to be repositioned in the orbit.

These eye movements are performed by the six extraocular muscles: superior rectus, inferior rectus, lateral rectus, medial rectus, lesser oblique and greater oblique muscles (Figure 10). They are innervated by the motor neurons of the oculomotor (nucleus III), trochlear (nucleus IV) and abducens (nucleus VI) nuclei. The motor neurons of the abducens (VI) and trochlear (IV) nuclei monosynaptically innervate a single muscle, the ipsilateral lateral rectus and contralateral oblique longus, respectively. In addition, the abducens nuclei consist of internuclear neurons whose axons cross the midline and project into the oculomotor nucleus (III), which innervates the medial rectus muscle. These internuclear neurons play an important role in the conjugate movements of the eyes. The oculomotor nucleus III innervates the following four muscles: on the ipsilateral side, the inferior rectus, the internal rectus and the lesser oblique muscle; and on the contralateral side, the superior rectus muscle.

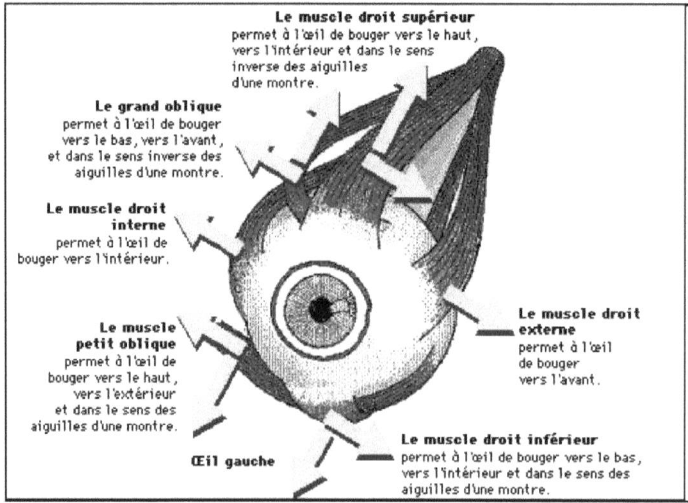

Figure 9: Representation of the oculomotor muscles

b/ Vestibulo-spinal system:

It participates in the stabilisation reactions of the head and body in space.

It is divided into three bundles that originate in the vestibular nuclei: the lateral vestibulospinal bundle (VSLB), the medial vestibulospinal bundle (MVB) and the caudal vestibulospinal bundle (CVB).

<u>The lateral vestibulospinal bundle :</u>

It originates from the lateral vestibular nucleus and is strictly ipsilateral. The fibres end in the grey matter of the ventral horn with cervical, thoracic and lumbar projection.

FVSL has facilitative effects on the alpha and gamma motor neurons of the extensor muscles.

These mono- and polysynaptic influences affect both the axial and distal muscles.

The afferents of the SLVF are of the following types: labyrinthine, somatosensory and cerebellar.

<u>The medial vestibulospinal bundle :</u>

It is derived from several nuclei: the medial, inferior and lateral vestibular nuclei and is bilateral. Most of its fibres terminate at the cervical level, some at the thoracic level and none project to the lumbar level.

This bundle carries mainly, but not exclusively, information of ampullary origin. It has both facilitating and inhibiting influences on the motor neurons of the neck and back muscles.

<u>The caudal vestibulospinal bundle :</u>

The FVSC is the least well known bundle. It originates from the caudal poles of the medial and descending nuclei. It descends bilaterally to the lumbar level. Their effect is mainly facilitative.

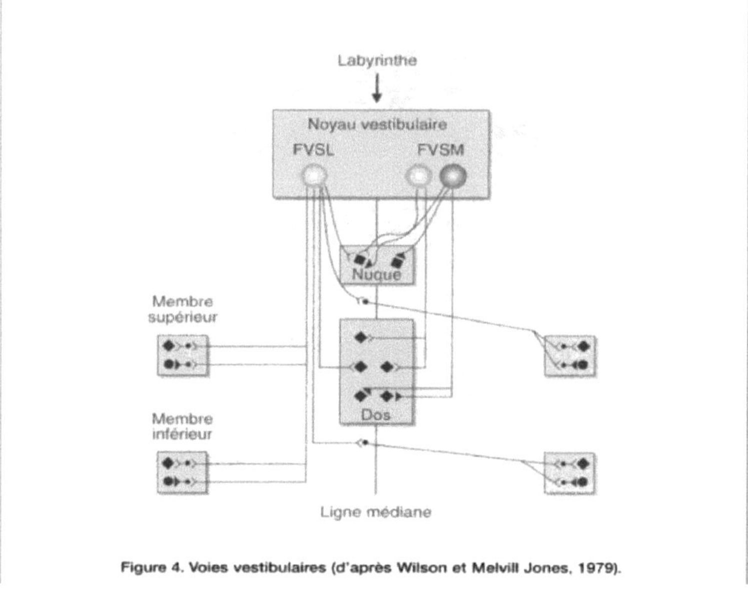

Figure 4. Voies vestibulaires (d'après Wilson et Melvill Jones, 1979).

<u>Figure 10:</u> Organisation of the vestibulo-spinal system

2-4: Vestibulo-cerebellar connections :

The vestibulo-cerebellar and cerebello-vestibular pathways coordinate movement with changes in posture.

The cerebellar cortex involved includes the flocculus, paraflocculus, nodulus and uvula. It is involved in the mechanisms of image stabilisation on the retina. The cerebellar vermis, on the other hand, is involved more specifically in oculomotricity (Figure 12).

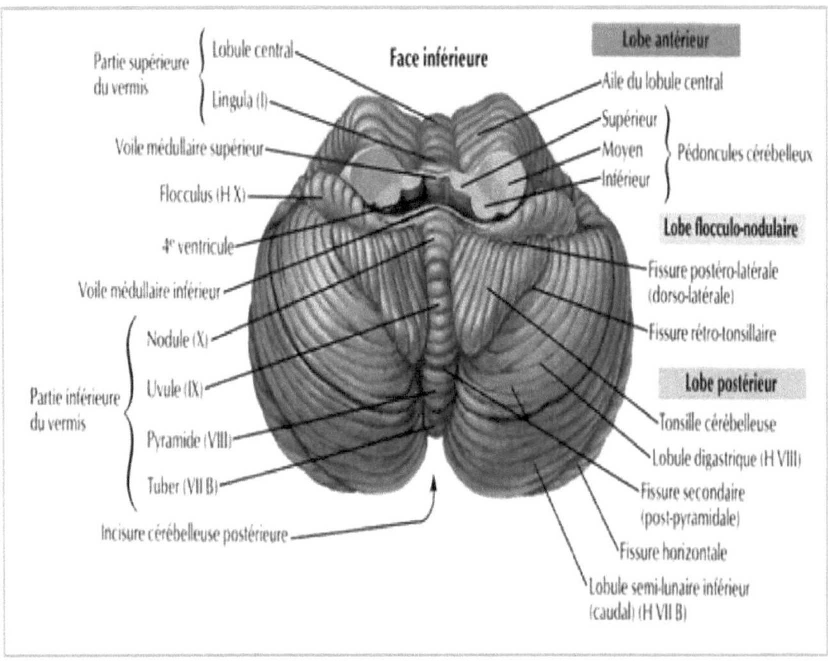

<u>Figure 11:</u> Representation of the cerebellum

The archaeocerebellum (flocculo-nodular lobe) receives vestibular information via the inferior cerebellar peduncle and controls it.

After relaying to the fastigial nucleus, the cerebellar efferences project via the inferior cerebellar peduncle to the vestibular nuclei, which send a coordinated motor command to the reticular formation and the ventral horns of the medulla.

The vestibular nuclei stimulate the nuclei of the ponto-mesencephalic reticular formation and through the ventral reticulo-spinal bundle activate the motor neurons, reinforcing the tone of the anti-gravidic muscles (Figure 13).

Thus, from the cerebellum there are direct and ipsilateral projections to the vestibular nuclei, the hypoglossal nucleus and also direct oculomotor and cortical projections.

- ARCHEO CEREBELLUM =
équilibre
- Pédoncules cérébelleux inf.
- N. vestibulaires + réticulés
du TC

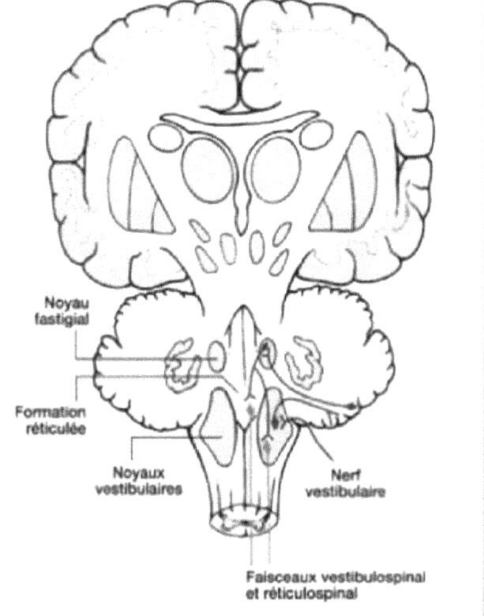

<u>Figure 12:</u> Representation of the vestibulo-cerebellar connections

2-5: Cortico-vestibular connections :

Recent work, particularly enhanced by the contribution of functional imaging, shows that the vestibular pathways project onto several cortical areas. In addition to this vestibular information, these areas also receive visual and proprioceptive information. Ultimately, the messages from the vestibular apparatus, which adjust the involuntary movements of the muscles of the eyes, head and body, are finally integrated with those of the visual and somaesthetic system by the cortex for a conscious perception of the position of the body in space.

CHAPTER 2

<u>*11- 2: Physiological reminders :*</u>

Balance is the stability of the body and the gaze despite changes in position or movement.

The balancing function requires three sources of information: ^vestibular

* visual

* proprioceptive.

These receptor systems conduct information to the central nervous system via afferent pathways. The effectors are represented by oculomotricity and the action of the antigravity muscles.

The lack of regulation of this system will result in a destabilization of the body and instability of the eyes, causing vertigo.

1 Physiology of labyrinthine receptors :

The functioning of the balance receptors is due to the fact that the bony labyrinth is rigid and moves with the body, whereas the membranous labyrinth contains fluids that can move according to the forces acting on them.

Each neuroepithelium is formed by 2 specialised cell types: type I cells and type II cells (Figure 14).

Their cilia, located at the upper pole of the cell, are composed of a single kinocil located at the periphery of a bundle of stereocilia.

Type I cells, which are amphora-shaped, have their cell bodies completely enclosed by the afferent vestibular fibres.

These type I cells are phasic, i.e. they respond only to movement of the ciliary tuft in the direction of cell polarisation.

Type II cells are rectangular in shape and synapse directly with the afferent and efferent nerve endings.

They are tonic, i.e. they discharge at rest and the mobility of the ciliary tuft will increase (in the direction of polarisation) or decrease (in the opposite direction) the electrical activity;

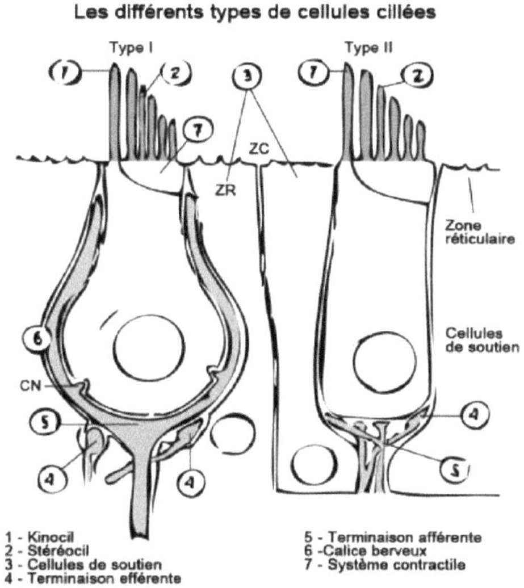

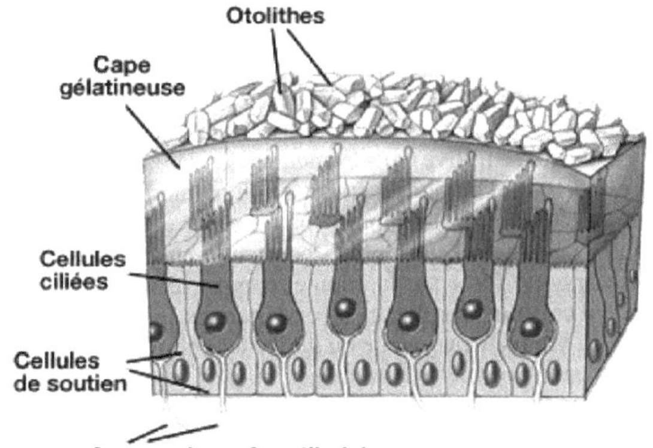

Figure 13: Representation of vestibular hair cells

1-1: Otolith macules :

These are the receptors of linear and gravitational displacement.

The two otolith maculae lie on perpendicular planes. Thus, the stimuli are mainly horizontal accelerations for the utricular receptors and vertical accelerations for the saccular receptors.

Their apical pole is formed by the tips of the cilia of the cells and is covered by a gelatinous membrane weighed down by the presence of otoconia (Figure 15).

Figure 14: Representation of the otolith macule

Each macule is divided into two equal areas by the striola. On each side of the striola, the cell polarisation vectors are reversed, so that all cells have their kinocils oriented on the side of the striola for the utricle and on the opposite side for the saccule. Thus, macular sensitivity is multidirectional (Figure 16).

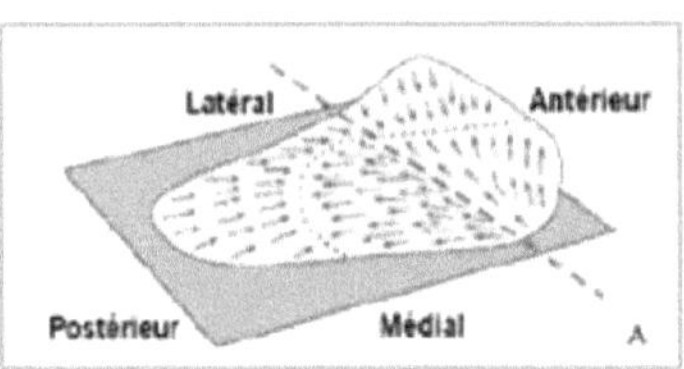

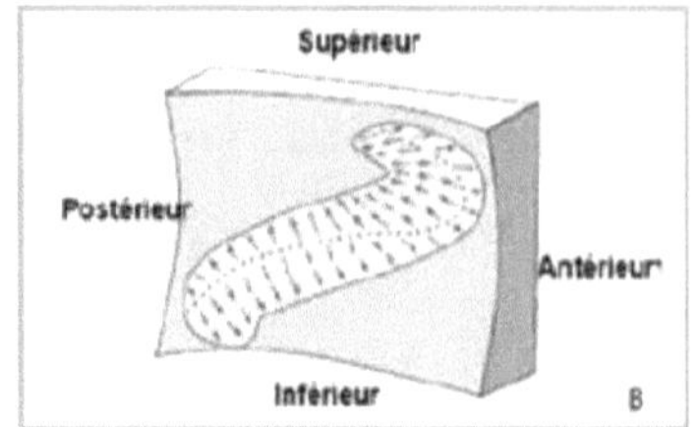

Figure 15: Orientation and polarisation of macules A: utricle, B: saccule

1-2: Ampullary ridges:

These are the neurosensory organs of the semicircular canals. They act as angular accelerometers.

The ampullary ridges lie in a plane perpendicular to that of the duct and represent one third of its height. They are surmounted by a protein-rich gelatinous structure, the cupula, which acts as an inertial mass in the ampullary ridge. The composition of the cupula is similar to that of the gelatinous layer of the otoconic membrane but there are no otoconia. All the cells of the same ridge are polarised in the same direction:

The ampulla (towards the ampulla) for the lateral canal, and the ampulla (towards the canal) for the posterior and anterior canals. Type I phasic cells are located at the top and type II cells at the base (Figure 17).

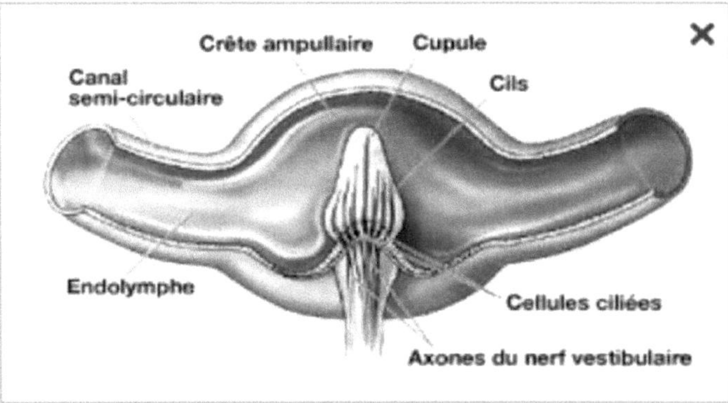

Figure 16: Representation of the ampullary ridge

1-3: Mechanotransduction :

The movement of the head is accompanied by a movement of the endolymphatic fluids, which leads to the movement of the ciliary tuft. These hair cells will transform a mechanical signal, the deflection of the ciliary tuft, into an electrical signal, i.e. generate action potentials on the afferent fibre. This is called mechanotransduction.

The first step in mechanotransduction is the deflection of the ciliary tuft in the direction of the kinocilium, which induces an elongation of the tip-links that allows the opening of the mechanotransduction channels and the entry of K+ and Ca2+ cations. The entry of cations creates an intracellular current that depolarises the cell: this defines the cell's

16

receptor potential. This depolarisation activates the voltage-dependent calcium channels. These channels open, the release of glutamate and the frequency of action potentials increase. The mechanotransduction channels, after opening, return to a closed, non-activatable and then activatable conformation. There is therefore a recovery time before reactivation. The opposite phenomenon occurs when the cilia bend in the opposite direction (Figure 7).

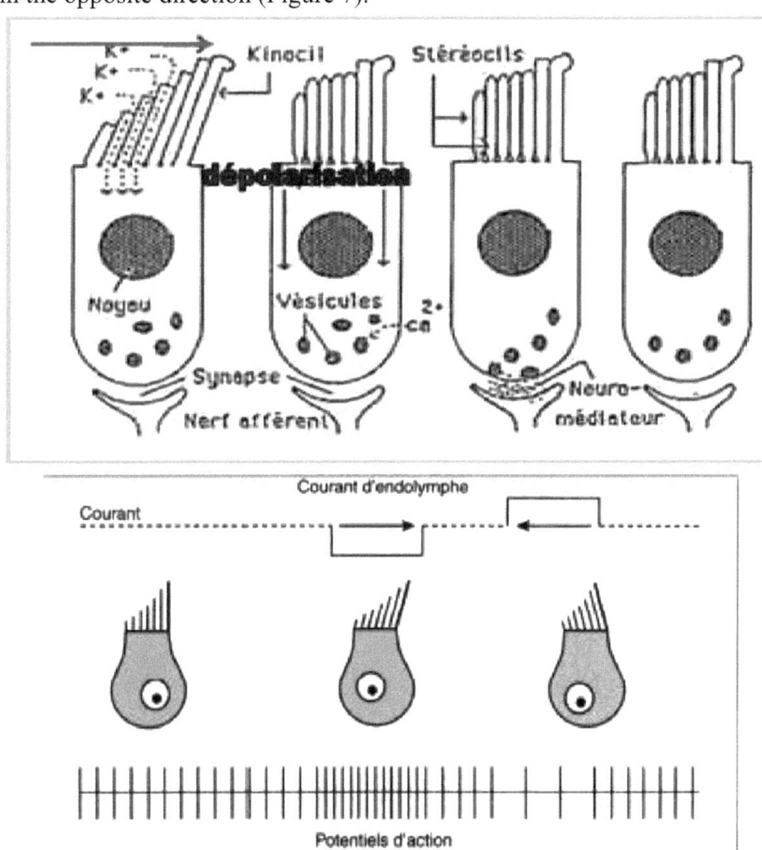

<u>Figure 17:</u> Representation of the mechanotransduction steps.

2 *Root canal :*

The semicircular canals serve to encode rotational accelerations. Endolymphatic movement in the canal causes deflection of the cup by the fluid stream and results in displacement of the ciliary tufts and depolarisation of the hair cells.

The information will be routed via the ampullary nerves to the superior vestibular nucleus and to the rostral part of the median vestibular nucleus. From there, very important pathways lead to the nuclei of the oculomotor muscles of the cerebellum, the motor neurons of the skeletal musculature and the postcentral gyrus (seat of conscious spatial orientation).

-Canalospinal pathways: These pathways follow the medial vestibulospinal bundle bilaterally and project preferentially to the cervical medulla. Generally speaking, canal stimulation leads to a postural reaction that facilitates cephalic displacement in compensation for the stimulation.

Stimulation of the horizontal canal activates the contralateral flexor muscles and inhibits the ipsilateral cervical muscles. Stimulation of the anterior channel activates the head extensor muscles and inhibits the flexors bilaterally. Stimulation of the posterior canal activates the flexor muscles and inhibits the extensors.

-Canalo-oculomotor pathways: induce a compensatory eye movement in the direction of the stimulated canal. It is a reflex arc with three neurons: primary and secondary vestibular and oculomotor motor neuron. Most of the canalo-oculomotor fibres run in the medial longitudinal bundle in an ascending, crossing (excitatory fibres) and non-crossing (inhibitory fibres) fashion.

Stimulation of the horizontal canal induces contraction of the contralateral lateral rectus and homolateral medial rectus muscles, as well as inhibition of their contralateral counterparts (Figure 18).

The vertical canals are connected to four muscles on each side: small and large obliques, inferior rectus and superior rectus. The contralateral anterior and posterior canals are coplanar and are activated by movements in opposite directions.

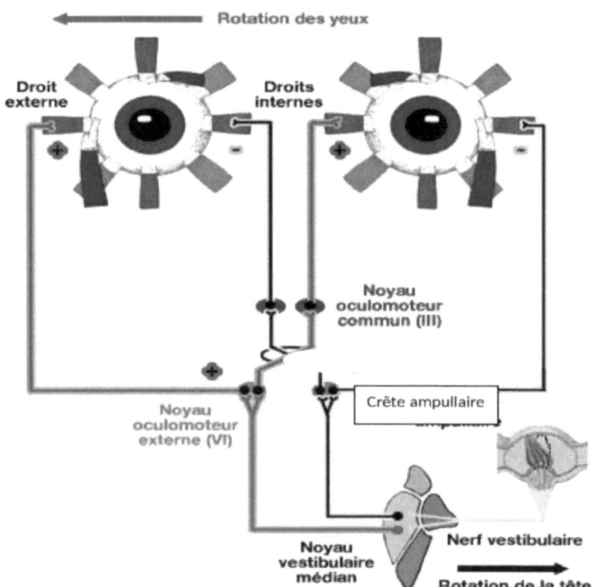

<u>Figure 18:</u> Canal-oculomotor pathways of the horizontal semicircular canals

3 Otolith pathways :

The otolith organs are responsible for the transduction of linear acceleration forces.

When the head is moved horizontally or tilted, the gelatinous layer will deflect the sensory cilia and cause mechanotransduction.

The utricular information will be conveyed via the superior vestibular nerve to the ventral part of the lateral vestibular nucleus in the bridge and the saccular information via the inferior vestibular nerve to the dorsolateral part of the inferior vestibular nucleus.

These afferents synapse with secondary vestibular neurons and a network of interneurons.

Secondary neurons of otolith origin project to four major systems: the medulla, oculomotor nuclei, cerebellum and cortex.

- Maculo-spinal pathways :

*The main role of the utriculospinal tracts is to maintain the head in relation to the trunk during horizontal acceleration. They pass through the ipsilateral FVSL.

*The sacculospinal tracts have a more accessory role of maintaining the head during vertical movements. They pass through the FVS, bilaterally, embedded in the canalicular afferents, and project to the cervical cord exclusively.

-Maculo-oculomotor pathways: Their purpose is to keep the retinal image stable during movement.

4-Efferent system

Efferent control, from the central nervous system, modulates afferent messages from the balance receptors. This feedback is provided by efferent synapses contacting either type II cells directly or the calyces of type I cells. The cell bodies of the efferent neurons come mostly from a nucleus adjacent to the vestibular nucleus in the brainstem, but also from Purkinje cells in the cerebellum. The activity of the efferent system is dependent on several sensory systems. At several levels, it is the afferent vestibular activity that regulates the efferents, but there is also control of the efferent pathways by visual and proprioceptive afferents. The predominant neurotransmitter in the efferent system is acetylcholine.

III-l: Interests of videonystagmography :

ENT doctors can examine the vestibular function by closely observing the eye movements and by focusing in particular on the rapid, involuntary movement known as "nystagmus". This nystagmus, although observed under Frenzel glasses, can only be analysed in 3 dimensions with its three horizontal, vertical and torsional components using VNG. VNG allows the detection of physiological or non-physiological eye movements, even the finest, in real time, to quantify them and thus to put forward a diagnostic hypothesis confronted with the clinical data. It can explore a whole range of frequencies between 0.001 and 100 Hz.

III-2: VNG scheme and principle :

The VNG consists of an infrared Charge Coupled Device (CCD, definition 320,000 pixels) camera mounted on a completely light-tight mask. This device is connected to a computer which digitises the analogue signal emitted by the pupil (Figure 19).

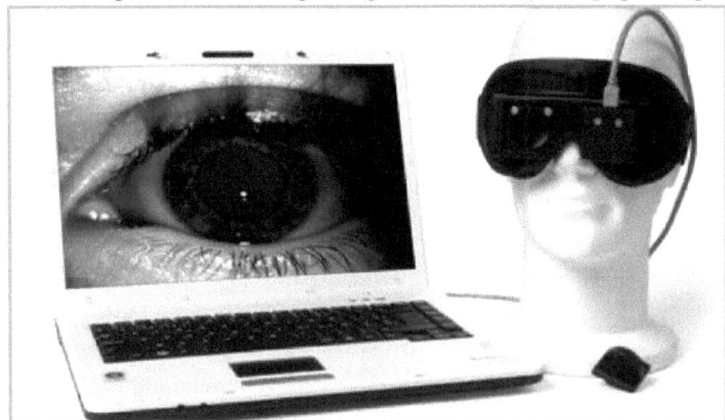

Figure 19: VNG device.

Only one eye is filmed, while the other can either access the scenery or be deprived of it at will, leaving both eyes in total darkness. To achieve this total darkness, the filmed eye is illuminated by diodes in the mask. The infrared radiation is outside the human visual spectrum. The principle is based on the detection of the iris print and thus to collect an image of the eye. The camera converts this image of the eye into a video signal. The video signal is then sent to a video acquisition card in the computer. This card converts the video signal into a sequence of bytes that it stores in the computer's memory. A pre-established program then performs the detection algorithm and calculates the position angles of the eye with reference to its centre. A calibration phase is therefore necessary. This operation consists of empirically establishing a relationship between a known angle of ocular deflection on the one hand and the amplitude of the corresponding deflection expressed as a number of points on the VNG plot on the other.

During subsequent examinations, the quality of the movements collected will depend on the correct performance of this phase, which is constant in the test subject (Figure 20).

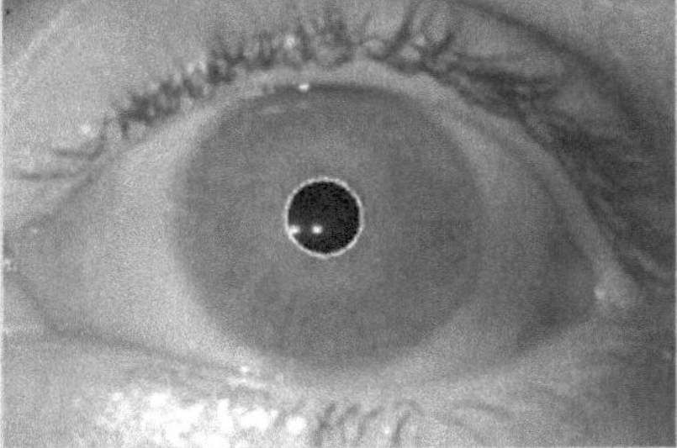

Figure 20: Detection and centring of the eye.

In addition to the mask and the microprocessor, a visualization device, water or air irrigation equipment and a rotating chair are required.

VNG usually records the movement of only one eye: the one on the camera side as a trace. The other eye is opened in the light with or without eye fixation, or placed in the dark with the help of a mask. The eye movements are recorded in the horizontal and vertical directions. For horizontal movement, the baseline represents the eye in the median position. If the eye moves to the right, the line bends upwards. If the eye moves to the left, the trace bends downwards. For the vertical movement recording, if the eye moves upwards, the trace bends upwards. If the eye moves downwards, the trace bends downwards. The slope of the curve represents the speed of eye movement (Figure 21). By convention, the direction of the nystagmus is that of the fast phase.

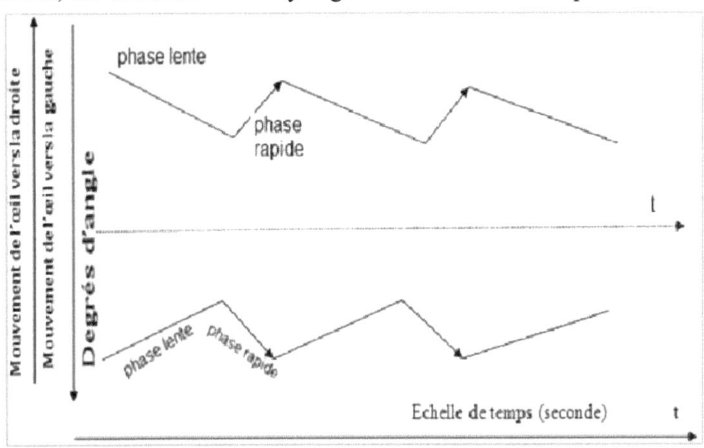

Figure 21: Interpretation of nystagmus directions.

III-3: Technique for carrying out the various tests and their results :

In practice, the examination is conducted in the following order:

- A calibration on the horizontal axis by asking the subject, whose head is straight and mobile, to stare alternately at targets arranged in his visual field. As the eye is quasi-spherical, it follows that the calibration performed in the horizontal axis is valid in the vertical axis.

- A study of gaze stability and oculomotricity.
- A recording of spontaneous and then induced nystagmus.
- Rotational kinetic tests.
- Caloric challenges.

III-3-1: Study of oculomotricity :

The various oculomotor tests are performed in a master-slave mode. The stimulated eye is called master and the recorded eye is called slave. This requires prior verification of the normality of the ocular conjugation of the two eyes and the sufficiency of the peripheral and central visions. The oculomotor tests are carried out by asking the subject to stare at a real target at a distance of about one metre to avoid eccentricity of gaze beyond 30°. The source is controlled by a computer. It can be fixed or be animated by a slow regular movement (pursuit test) or jump from one position to another (saccadic tests).

1/ Slow eye-tracking test:

The subject must follow a visual target that moves slowly in the horizontal plane from right to left and left to right, or in the vertical plane from top to bottom and bottom to top. This is a sinusoidal stimulation of 0.4 Hz, with an amplitude of plus or minus 20° in the horizontal plane and 27° in the vertical plane.

in the vertical plane. The eye sticks to the target. Eye tracking is quickly disrupted and disorganised by fatigue, visual impairment and ageing.

The general appearance of the curve obtained must be smooth, with an absence of saccadic phenomena. These are found in central syndromes (Figure 22).

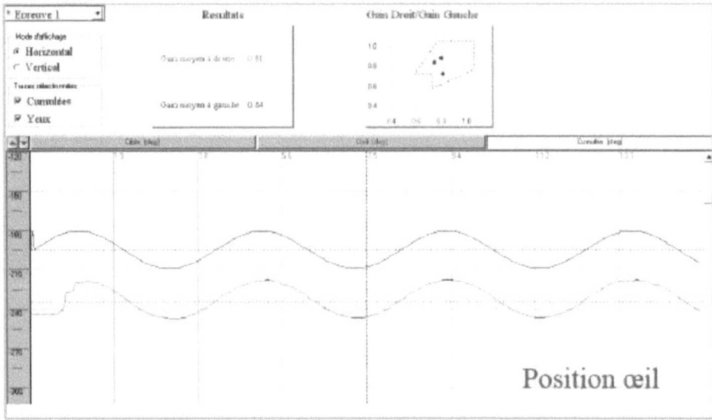

<u>Figure 22:</u> Horizontal slow eye tracking in a normal subject: green is the visual stimulation and red is the eye movement. The gain is greater than 0.7 and is symmetrical.

§ The gain of these tracking movements (ratio of eye speed to target speed) is then automatically calculated and compared to pre-set standards. In peripheral pathologies and in normal subjects, this parameter should be greater than 0.7 and symmetrical. Lesions of the cerebellum as well as central pathologies and drugs decrease the gain of the tracking system. In internuclear ophthalmoplegia, the gain is collapsed and the eye movements are dysconjugate: the pursuit movements of the right eye are not superimposable to the pursuit movements of the left eye (Figure 23).

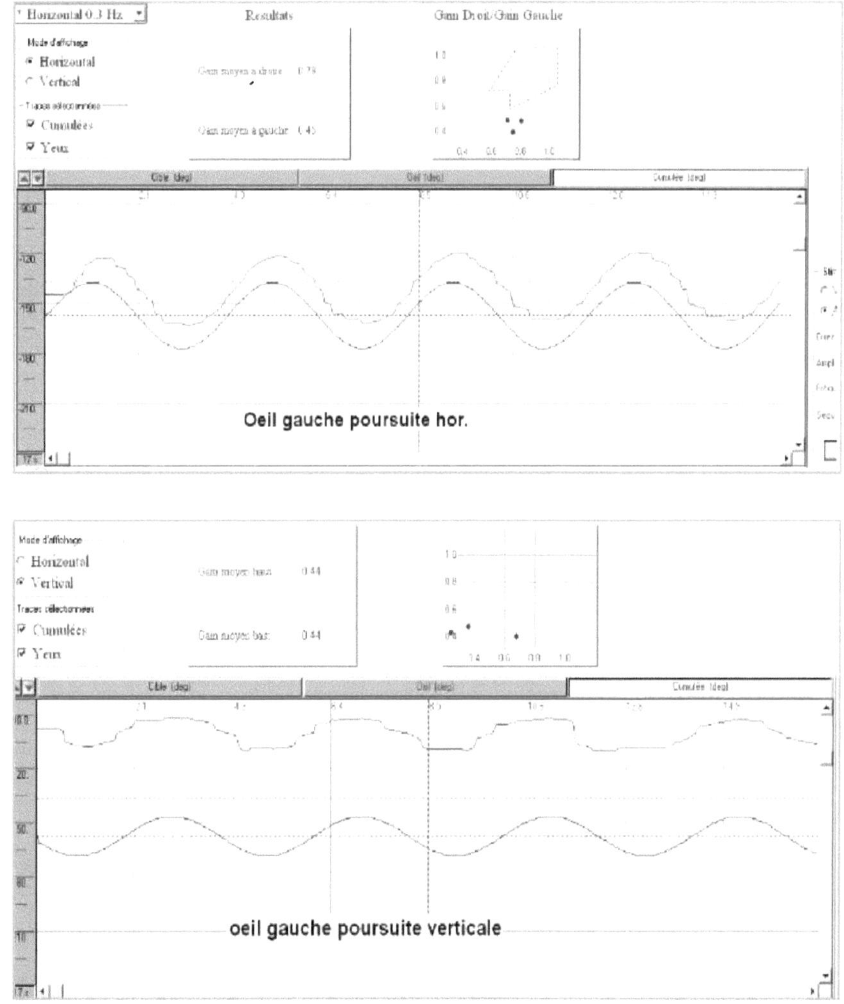

Figure 23: Horizontal and vertical slow eye tracking patterns in a subject with internuclear ophthalmoplegia. In red the eye movement and in green the target movement. The gain is

collapsed and asymmetric.

<u>**2/ Saccade test:**</u>

Visual attraction saccades are triggered reflexively when a target appears at the periphery of the retina. Most subjects make a first saccade, known as a refixation saccade, the amplitude of which is 90% of the final amplitude, followed by a second correction saccade after a latency of about 130 ms.

The study of saccades can be done using a totally random or non-random sequence with a maximum amplitude of +/- 20°.

§ Regular sequence: the test starts with the fixation of a point of light which appears in the middle of the screen. Once the sequence has started, the fixation point disappears and reappears either on the right or on the left with an angulation of 20°. During the 35-second test period, the dot alternates between the right and left sides of the screen with a regular frequency of 0.30 Hz, without returning to the central position. This sequence is thus characterised by a predictable onset time and target location. The saccades are regular.

§ Random sequence: the test is characterised by a predictable target location, defined by its magnitude and direction, but with temporal uncertainty, the sequence being temporally random.

We will analyse :

1) <u>*Refixation latency is*</u> defined as the delay (in milliseconds) between stimulus onset and ocular response. Many factors influence latencies: age, fatigue, training, sedative drugs and the predictability of the stimulus. It is less than 250 ms for healthy subjects and in peripheral pathologies and is increased in central pathologies.

2) <u>*Accuracy*</u> is the ratio of the amplitude of the refixation saccade to the angle of deflection of the target, and its normal value is between 70 and 100%. Accuracy is controlled by the cerebellum. Hypometry is defined by an accuracy < 75% and hypermetry by an accuracy > 100%. Hypermetria is quite exceptional and is seen in internuclear ophthalmoplegia (Figure 24) and in Wallenberg syndrome. Hypometria is a sign frequently encountered in cerebellar disorders (saccade speed is normal) and in brainstem disorders (degenerative demyelinating disease, Friedrich's disease, Parkinson's disease), often associated with a slowing down. Finally, parietal damage is accompanied by a hypometry of saccades in the contralateral direction.

3) <u>*The maximum speed of the saccade*</u> is a direct function of the amplitude. For an amplitude of 40°, the maximum speed reaches 400° / sec. This measurement is important because it can reveal sub-clinical oculomotor paresis. For example, a left external oculomotor nerve (VI) injury will result in a slowing down of the saccadic velocities of the left eye when looking to the left. The slowing of saccades is also of great clinical interest in intrinsic brainstem damage: degenerative, demyelinating, tumour or vascular.

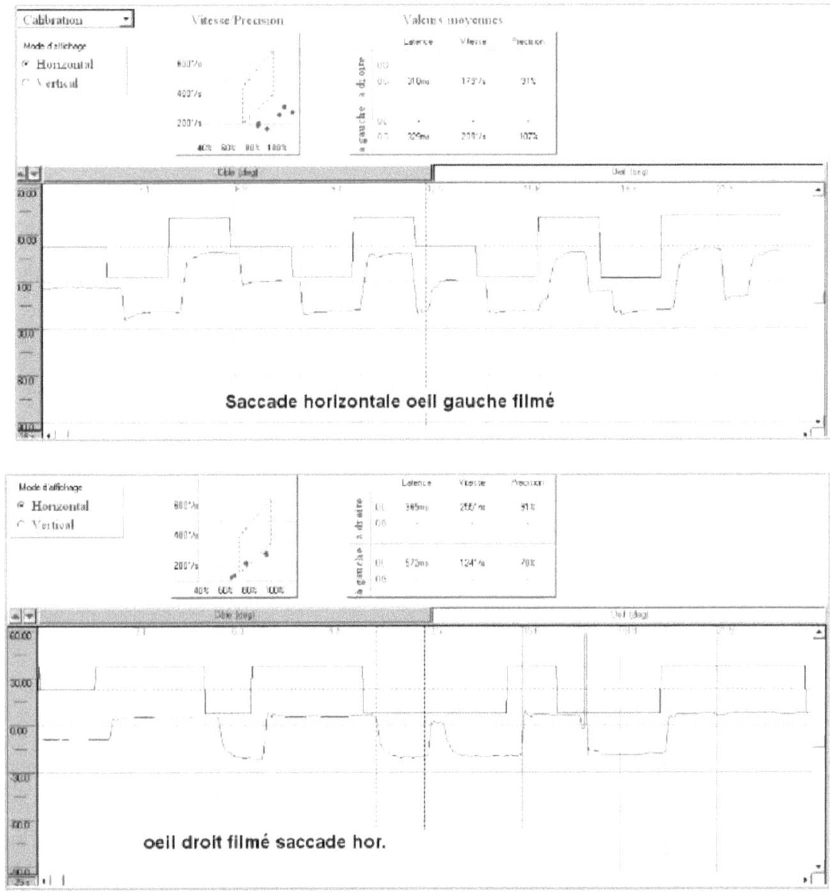

Saccade horizontale oeil gauche filmé

oeil droit filmé saccade hor.

<u>Figure 24:</u> Saccade patterns of both eyes in a subject with internuclear ophthalmoplegia. In red the eye movement and in green the target movement. Latency and accuracy are high.

3/ Optokinetic nystagmus:

The optokinetic reflex (OKR) is an ocular stabilisation reflex that is triggered by the rotation of the environment as a whole and is intended to reduce retinal slippage.

There are two central channels of the optokinetic system:

*A cortical pathway that uses the pursuit system (the subject looks attentively); the latency is short (100 ms), the gain is close to 1 for a stimulus speed between 30 and 507sc then collapses for a higher speed.

* a subcortical pathway (accessory optic system); the latency is long, the gain is low with a clear retinal shift and an optokinetic post-nystagmus of the same direction as the optokinetic nystagmus. It is this system that is most involved in visuovestibular interaction and the production of sensations such as vection. Stimulation of this

pathway can be achieved by asking the subject to look into the blur.

In practice, the subject must be situated in front of a field that is usually wide and on which black and white stripes or luminous dots (optokinetic ball) are projected, which can scroll in the horizontal or vertical plane. The speed of the stimulation is constant and can vary between 10 and 807s. The subcortical optokinetic nystagmus pathway is explored by the vague gaze and the pursuit system by the fixed gaze. Unilateral peripheral vestibular lesions result in a decrease in the gain of the optokinetic reflex for stimuli directed towards the side of the lesion. These gain asymmetries decrease over time (Figure 25).

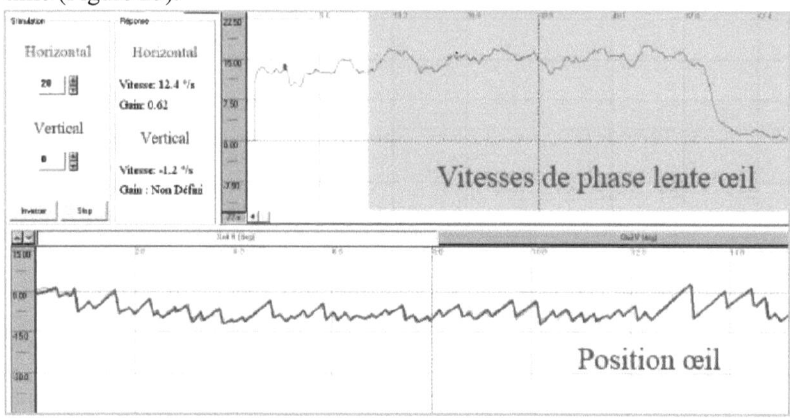

Figure 25: Plot of normal optokinetic nystagmus

III-3-2: Study of spontaneous nystagmus :

Spontaneous nystagmus is defined as nystagmus observed with the head upright, in gaze not exceeding an excursion of 30° (the inner edge of the iris of the eye opposite to the required movement should not be allowed to reach the coruncle), in the absence of a foveal fixation cue. This position must be stable for a sufficient time (two minutes) to eliminate the influence of a recent change in position. The minimum observation time is 30 seconds.

The subject is seated, head upright and motionless in a stable environment. The recording is first performed in the light with the master eye uncovered, then in the dark with the master eye covered by a mask. Whether the subject is in the light or in the dark, the search for spontaneous nystagmus is carried out in the direction of the primary gaze: the gaze straight ahead or median, then by asking the subject to move the gaze to the right, then to the left, and upwards, without exceeding 30°.

*In the normal subject there should be no spontaneous nystagmus (Figure 26).

Sometimes, square waves of ocular instability of low amplitude (0.5 to 5°) can be recorded. They are usually of no pathological value. They can be found in the elderly, in cases of progressive supranuclear palsy, strabismus, and focal brain lesions. They have been described in chorea and schizophrenia. Other abnormal movements are:

opsoclonus, flutter...

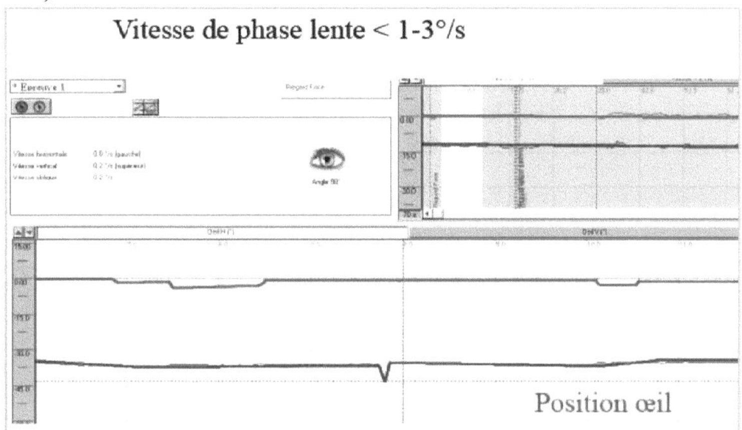

Figure 26: Search for spontaneous nystagmus: absent in this subject

* The presence of spontaneous nystagmus is pathological. It is characterised by its type, direction, intensity and whether or not it is influenced by fixation.

The type :

Pendular nystagmus: consists of two jerks of equal duration and amplitude. It is therefore not possible to define a direction (Figure 27).

There is congenital and acquired pendular nystagmus.

-Idiopathic congenital nystagmus is defined by the presence of spontaneous, bilateral, involuntary, oscillatory movements of the eyeballs, present from birth or appearing during the first three months of life. These nystagmus jerks persist throughout life. Nystagmus twitches are often symmetrical and usually beat horizontally in 95% of patients. They may persist when the eyes are closed. However, idiopathic congenital nystagmus tends to subside during non-visual tasks. The pathophysiology of idiopathic congenital nystagmus remains poorly understood, but it is thought to be due to an abnormality in oculomotor control. All modes of inheritance (autosomal, autosomal recessive, and dominant X-linked, recessive X-linked) have been described. The gene located on chromosome 6pl2 (NYS2) is involved in autosomal dominant forms. Genes located at Xpll.4-pll.3 (NYSl) and Xq26-q27 are associated with the different forms of X-linked nystagmus.

-Acquired pendular nystagmus usually has a vertical and torsional component of the same frequency as the horizontal frequency. Its trajectory is oblique if the horizontal and vertical components are in phase; elliptical otherwise. It may be purely monocular and coexist with a tremor of other parts of the body, then resembling myoclonus. It can be found in cerebellar disorders, or associated with internuclear ophthalmoplegia, particularly in multiple sclerosis, brainstem vascular accidents, amblyopia or chiasma gliomas.

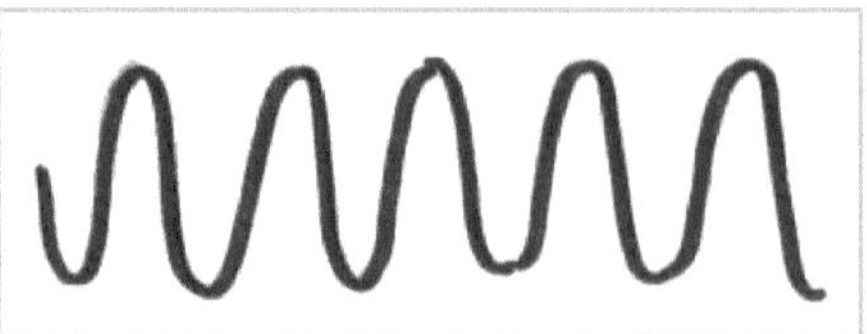

Spring nystagmus: has two phases of unequal duration, a slow phase and a fast phase. The fast phase defines the direction of the nystagmus (Figure 28).

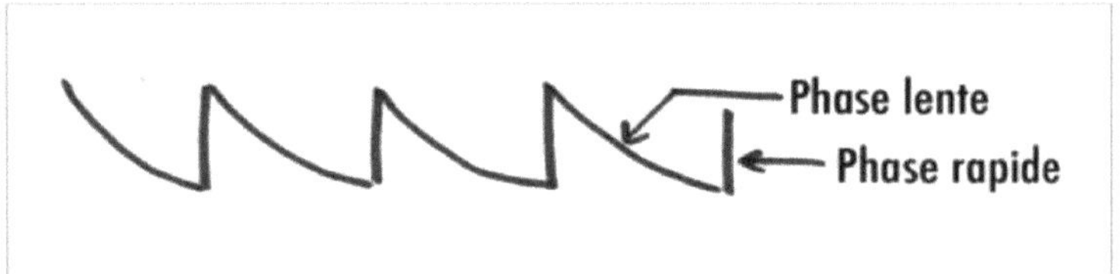

Meaning :

In spring nystagmus, the direction is that of the rapid phase. It may be unidirectional or multidirectional.

Alternating nystagmus is of central origin and is seen in cerebellar disorders. The nystagmus beats in one direction for one to two minutes, then decreases, disappears and after an interval of 10 to 30 seconds and without any movement, reappears and beats in the opposite direction.

Direction: horizontal, vertical or horizontal-rotating.

Pure vertical nystagmus is often of central origin, indicating posterior fossa pathology or Arnold Chiari malformation.

Vertical nystagmus of peripheral origin is seen when both anterior or both posterior semicircular canals are affected.

Pure rotatory nystagmus is rarely seen and is of central origin in relation to nuclear damage.

Slow phase speed :

The evolution of the velocity of the slow phases is provided by the horizontal and vertical velocity acquisition curve.

Intensity* :

Alexander classification :

> Grade I: Nystagmus is only observed when the gaze is directed in the direction of the saccade.
>
> Grade II: I+ central gaze = spontaneous nystagmus
>
> Degree III: II+looking in the direction of the slow phase.

Influence of eye fixation :

It differentiates between peripheral and central involvement.

The nystagmus observed during gaze eccentricity (less than 30°) corresponds to gaze nystagmus. A symmetrical horizontal gaze nystagmus is a sign of damage to the cerebellar flocculus or to the medial vestibular nuclei or of hypnotic, sedative or anxiolytic drugs.

Dissociated nystagmus gas is seen in internuclear ophthalmoplegia.

<u>Amplitude :</u>

Conjugate nystagmus with equal amplitude in both eyes is often peripheral.

A dissociated nystagmus predominantly in the abductor eye is of central origin.

In peripheral vestibular disease, spontaneous nystagmus has the following characteristics (Figure 29):

- ❖ A spring, with a conjugated character.
- ❖ Horizontal or horizontorotataory, is never purely vertical;
- ❖ diminished or abolished by ocular fixation
- ❖ increases when the gaze is directed to the side of the fast phase and decreases when looking at the opposite side.
- ❖ unidirectional and does not change direction in different gaze positions.

In central pathology, spontaneous nystagmus has the following characteristics:

- ❖ May be pendulous, no direction
- ❖ Alternating or multi-sensory
- ❖ Vertical, horizontal or purely rotational
- ❖ Multidirectional
- ❖ Not inhibited or increased by fixation
- ❖ Nystagmus gas in the eccentric gaze
- ❖ Dissociated

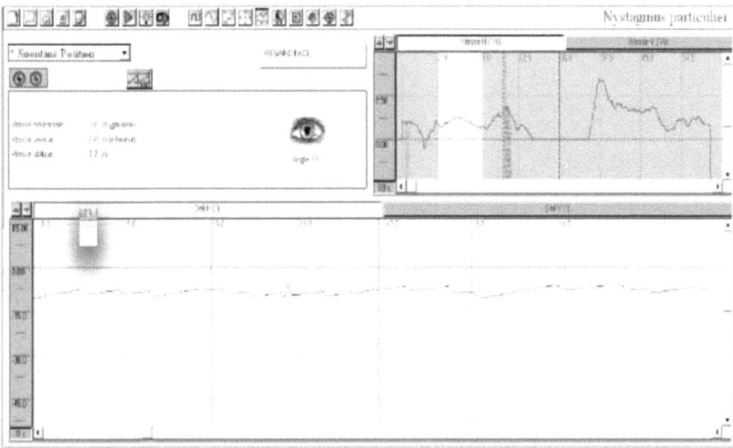

Figure 29: Spontaneous left horizontal nystagmus in right vestibular neuritis

III-3-3: Nystagmus induced by the Head Shaking Test:

The Head Shaking Test (HST) is an old, qualitative test that looks for vestibular asymmetry. It tests the reactivity of the two lateral channels at a frequency of 2 to 3 Hz. This activation generates a post-rotatory nystagmus thanks to the central velocity storage integrator. The principle is simple: a passive and symmetrical shaking of the head at 2Hz in a horizontal plane from left to right and from right to left for 20 seconds. When the stimulation is stopped, the potentially induced eye movements are analysed.

Symmetrical vestibular activity does not result in postrotatory nystagmus. Asymmetry reveals it in the form of a nystagmus with a rapid jerk beating on the side of the healthy ear.

This is the primary phase. It is followed by a secondary nystagmus of much longer duration (more than 60 seconds: secondary phase) whose fast phase beats on the injured side.

The induced nystagmus is horizontal in the case of a peripheral lesion (Figure 30) and is disharmonious or vertical in direction in the case of a central origin.

The Head Shaking Test can also reveal central anomalies in the speed storage integrator.

Importantly, it is a non-compensation sensitive test.

It is poorly tolerated in people with cervical osteoarthritis.

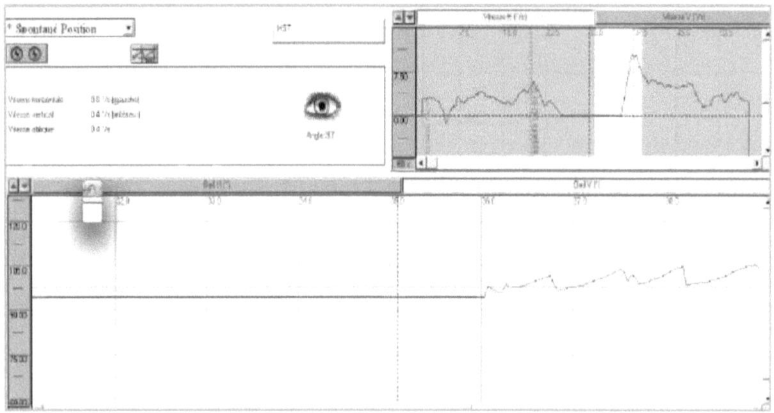

Figure 30: HST-induced left horizontal nystagmus in right vestibular neuritis

III-3-4: Positional Nystagmus:

Positional nystagmus is nystagmus caused by a change in head orientation. It is most often a sign of benign paroxysmal positional vertigo (BPPV).

BPPV is related to the presence of otoconial debris deposited on the cup of the labyrinthine vestibule (Cupulolithiasis Theory) or freely circulating in the semicircular canals (Canalolithiasis Theory) (Figure 31).

The triggering position and direction of the nystagmus determine which ear and canal are involved.

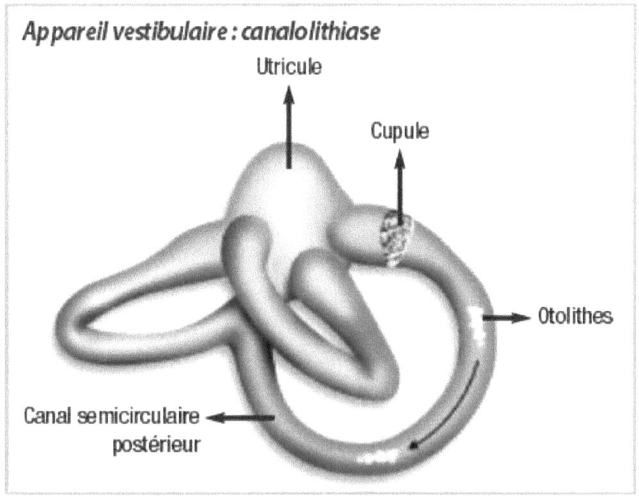

<u>Figure 31:</u> Representation of otoliths detached from macules

The diagnosis of <u>posterior canal BPPV is </u>based on the demonstration of typical nystagmus during the Dix-Hallpike manoeuvre. This manoeuvre consists of turning the patient's head 45° in the sitting position and tilting it backwards with the head extended 30° from the horizontal. The nystagmus appears after a minimum latency of one second, and is associated with vertigo. It is an upper vertical and geotropic, exhaustible nystagmus which reverses on change of position (Figure 32).

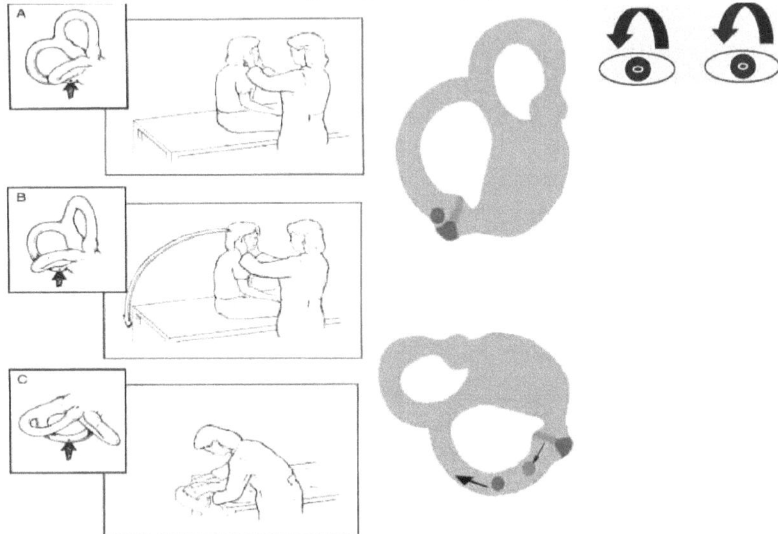

<u>Figure 32:</u> Dix and Hallpike manoeuvre for BPPV of the right posterior semicircular canal

<u>Lateral canal BPPV :</u>

Two forms are identified: geotropic and agetropic.

Geotropic form :

When placed in the triggering position with the head elevated 30°, the nystagmus is right horizontal in right rotation and the nystagmus is left horizontal in left rotation. The canalolithiasis theory is the most plausible (Figure 33).

Agiotropic form

When placed in the triggering position, with the head elevated by 30°, the nystagmus is left for a right rotation and right for a left rotation. The theory of cupulolithiasis is evoked.

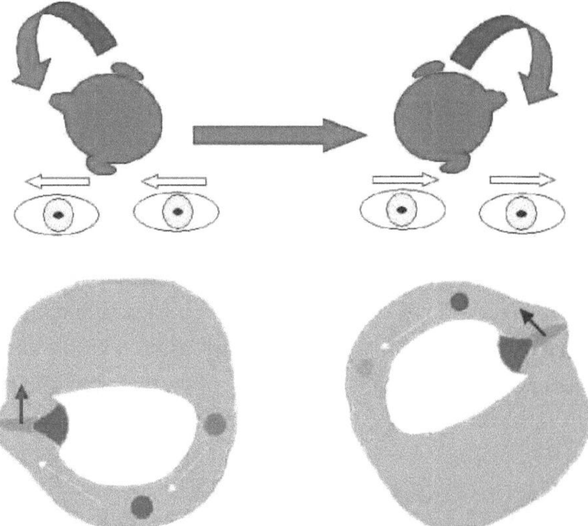

<u>Figure 33:</u> Diagnostic manoeuvre for BPPV of the left lateral semicircular canal: geotropic form.

<u>Anterior canal BPPV:</u>

This is a very rare clinical form. The diagnosis is made when a rotatory nystagmus with an inferior vertical component is detected after the Dix and Hallpike manoeuvre.

Some positional nystagmus is of central origin. Involvement of the dorsolateral part of the bulb and the dorsal part of the vermis is often incriminated.

Central positional nystagmus appears without a latency phase, is purely vertical or torsional, of prolonged duration, multidirectional and multisensory, not inhibited by fixation, not reversed on return to the sitting position, not fatiguable and does not follow any directional logic or evolutionary profile that could link it to canalolithiasis of a canal.

III-3-5: Rotational tests :

In everyday life, the accuracy of the correspondence between eye and head rotation speed is dependent on three sensory inputs: visual, vestibular and cervical proprioceptive. Kinetic tests allow the analysis of the ocular response, under physiological conditions, following the variation of one or more sensory inputs. They allow us to explore the medium frequencies (0.01-5Hz) which correspond to the frequencies of everyday life.

In practice, the subject sits in a chair that rotates around a vertical axis. The subject's head is tilted forward by 30° so that the horizontal CSCs are in a horizontal plane and the eye movements are recorded.

Different types of rotational stimulation can be performed: damped sinusoidal (gyratory pendulum test), frequency swept sinusoidal, impulse, and eccentric rotations. They study eye movements:

*With a visible decoration, this is the vestibulovisuoocular reflex,

*In total darkness it is the vestibulo-ocular reflex,

When the body turns but the head remains still, in the dark it is the oculocervical reflex,

*and with a stable visual reference that follows the movement of the chair - the visual fixation index (VFI).

Each type of kinetic stimulation interrogates the vestibule at different frequencies. The phase shift between cup deformation and head movement is zero between 0.1 and 5 Hz. There is a phase lead below (the deformation precedes the head movement) and a phase lag above (cup deformation lags behind the head movement). As a result, the gain is constant between 0.1 and 5 Hz and decreases for higher and lower frequencies (Figure 34).

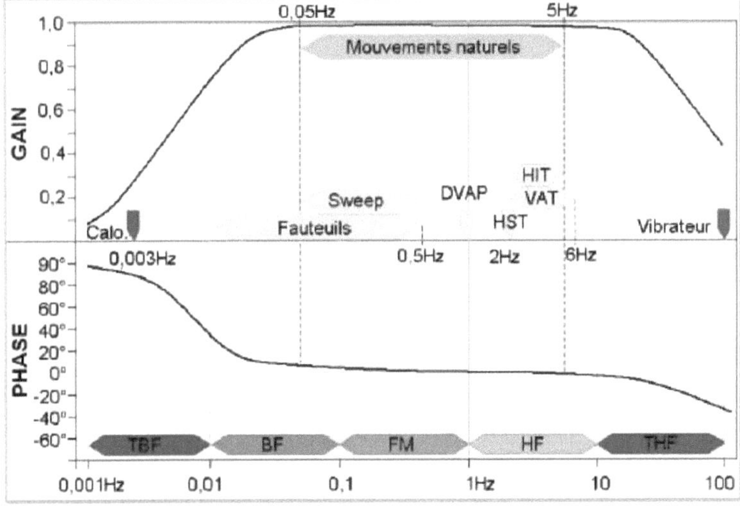

Figure 34: Representation of vestibular exploration areas

1- Horizontal sinusoidal rotations.

a/ Damped sinusoidal pendulum test :

It interrogates the vestibular system at a frequency of 0.05 Hz. The parameter studied is the average speed of the slow phase of the nystagmus. This is obtained by adding the slow phases and removing the fast phases of the nystagmus.

The cumulative plot is then shaped like a sinusoid that can be superimposed on the movement of the chair (Figure 35).

The gain (the ratio of eye speed to chair speed normally around 0.6), the preponderance (the asymmetry of the response to symmetrical stimulation normally <27sc), the phase shift (the offset between stimulation and eye movement normally 10°) and the time constant (the time after which the nystagmus decreases by 2/3 at around 20 seconds) are calculated (Figure 36).

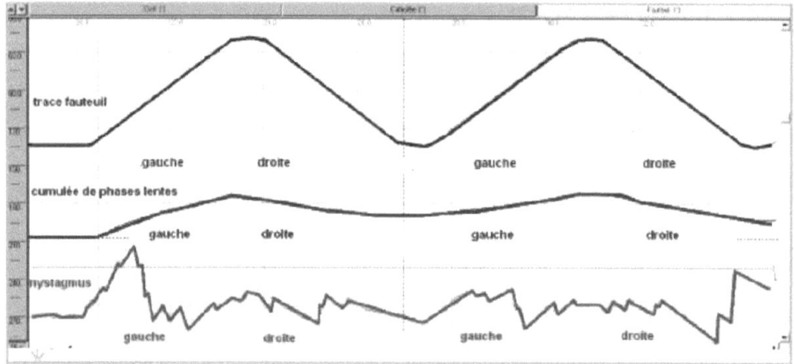

Figure 35: Representation of responses to sinusoidal stimulation Eye position plot: top ^ to the right, bottom ^ to the left Cumulative slow and armchair phase plots: top^ to the left, bottom ^ to the right

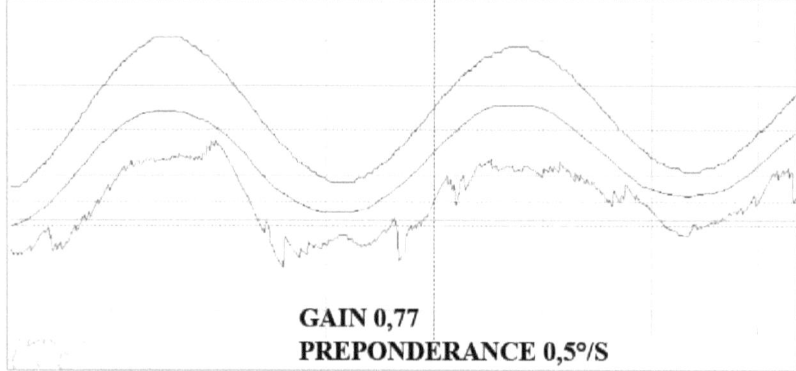

Figure 36: Representation of responses to sinusoidal stimulation

The index of inhibition of nystagmus by ocular fixation (IFO) is also studied in this test. In this case, the subject is asked to fixate a light target placed in the VNG mask while being rotated. Ocular fixation induces an inhibition of more than 50% of the horizontal vestibulo-ocular reflex gain in the normal subject. An IFO of less than 50%

is always indicative of central vestibular disease, but it has no precise localizing value. In the case of acute, unilateral labyrinth destruction, there is a bilateral decrease in gain, which is greater for rotations on the injured side than for rotations on the healthy side. At a distance, these abnormalities usually disappear due to central vestibular compensation.

b/ Frequency sweep sinusoidal pendulum test:

It allows the vestibular response to be analysed over a wider frequency range. In this test, the patient is placed on a chair with a sinusoidal movement whose period gradually shifts over 2 minutes from 20 to 2 seconds, corresponding to a frequency shift of 0.05 Hz to 0.5 Hz (Figure 37). The purpose of this test is to look for vestibular remnants in the case of bilateral areflexia as shown by the low frequency tests and to conclude that there is bilateral areflexia.

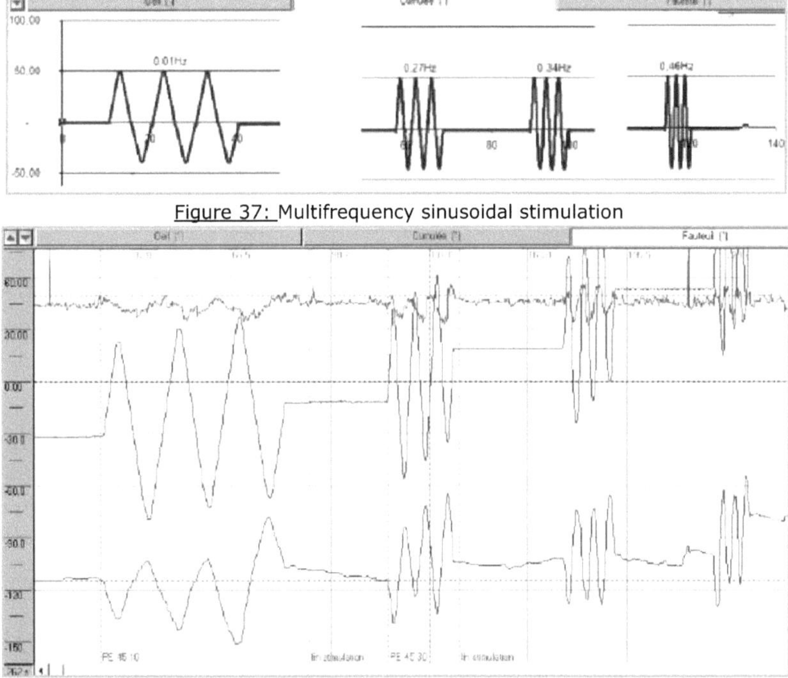

Figure 37: Multifrequency sinusoidal stimulation

Figure 37: Representation of tracings during multifrequency sinusoidal stimulation

2- Impulse tests

Alternatively, patients may be subjected to an acceleration of large amplitude followed by rotation at constant speed for 1 minute and finally deceleration of the same amplitude as the initial acceleration. In this case, we are interested in the nystagmus that occurs at the end of the rotation, the horizontal postrotatory nystagmus, and its disappearance time constant. It is about 20 seconds. It results from the activation of the velocity storage mechanism. After damage to the ampulla or the horizontal canal nerve, there is a greater bilateral decrease in the time constant of the reflex during rotations on the injured side than during rotations on the healthy side. This test is not sensitive to compensation (Figure 38).

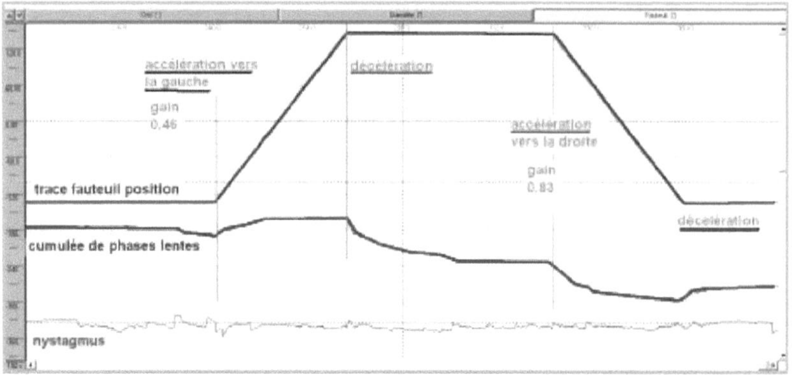

Figure 38: Representation of the traces during an impulse test

III-3-6: Caloric tests :

Described more than a century ago, this test is still relevant today. It allows the exploration of horizontal channels at very low frequency (0.005 Hz).

1/ Unilateral proof :

With the patient lying down, trunk raised by 30°, the test consists of successively irrigating the external auditory canals one by one with hot (44°C) then cold (30°C) water. The warm stimulation leads to an excitatory ampullipetic fluid movement and the cold stimulation to an inhibitory amuplifugal movement. The imbalance between the right and left activities results in a reflex nystagmus beating on the side opposite the cold stimulation and on the side of the warm stimulation. Irrigation is maintained for 30 seconds and the response is recorded between 60 and 90ème seconds after the start of stimulation, with 5 minutes of rest between the 2 stimulations.

In case of tympanic perforation, stimulation can be done with air (27 and 47°).

b/ Bilateral tests :

In this test, both ears are irrigated simultaneously. In the normal subject, this stimulation does not induce any nystagmus. In the pathological subject, a horizontal ocular nystagmus is observed. The direction of the rapid phase induced by the cold stimulation indicates the pathological side. This test is more sensitive than the unilateral test but also technically more difficult to perform.

Before any test, a bilateral otoscopic examination is necessary to eliminate a mechanical obstacle. The absence of an oculomotor problem must be ascertained. Certain drugs with a vestibuloplegic effect must be stopped 2 to 8 days beforehand, depending on the duration of life, e.g. neuroleptics, antihistamines, anxiolytics and barbiturates. Alcohol has a disinhibiting effect. Antivertiginous drugs with a long half-life (Flunarizine) must be stopped 15 days before. Acetylleucine can be tolerated.

The analysis of the nystagmus induced by caloric stimulation is done on an acquisition window that provides (Figure 39):

- 3 charts :

*The Freyss butterfly in maximum speed of the slow phase and in frequency of nystagmus.

*the radish graph: curve of evolution of slow phase velocities.

*The fir tree: recording of spontaneous eye movement and after each stimulation.

-values: reflectivity, prominence and deficit (see definitions below).

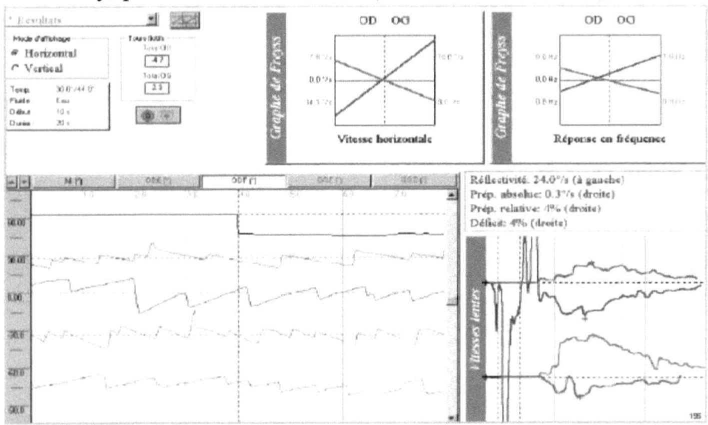

Figure 39: Representation of the results of a caloric test.

The directional preponderance

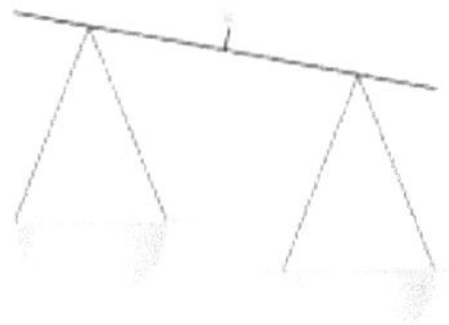

The vestibular stimulation can be of any nature, kinetic or caloric: the important thing is that it is symmetrical.

▶ Vestibular reflectivity

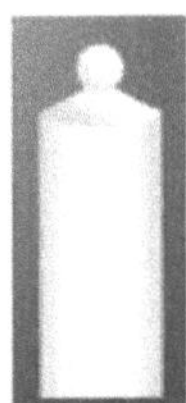

Vestibular reflectivity is the ability of the vestibule, whether in isolation or in pairs, to respond to a given stimulus. The concept of reflectivity therefore implies a simultaneous knowledge of the stimulation and the response. Depending on whether or not response and stimulation can be measured in the same unit, the numerical expression of reflectivity will vary.

► Hypovalence

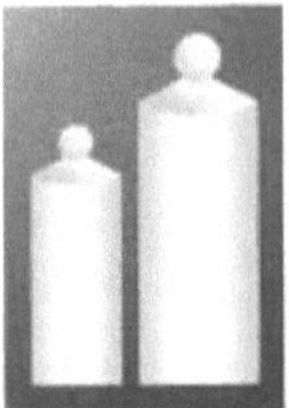

Hypovalence reflects the sensory deficit of one vestibule compared to the other. Because of the need to separate the two vestibules to make such a comparison, the term hypovalence is practically reserved for caloric tests only.

Interpretation (Figures 40, 41 and 42):

* The absolute reflectivity is the sum of the warm and cold responses for each ear. It ranges from 30 to 120 shocks. It is important to compare this value with the value of the opposite side.

* the relative reflectivity represents the notion of respective symmetry of the 2 vestibules. It represents the ratio of the sum of the responses of the left labyrinth to those of the right labyrinth. It is normally less than 15%.

* the directional dominance represents the predominant direction of the nystagmus response. It is obtained by comparing the sum of the straight nystagmus responses to the sum of the warm nystagmus responses. The ratio is normally less than 11%.

In the Freyss caloric test diagram, the right ear responses are plotted on the right vertical axis, the left ear responses on the left vertical axis. Left-beating nystagmus is plotted on the lower part of the diagram and right-beating nystagmus on the upper part. In a normal subject, a butterfly-like appearance is obtained.

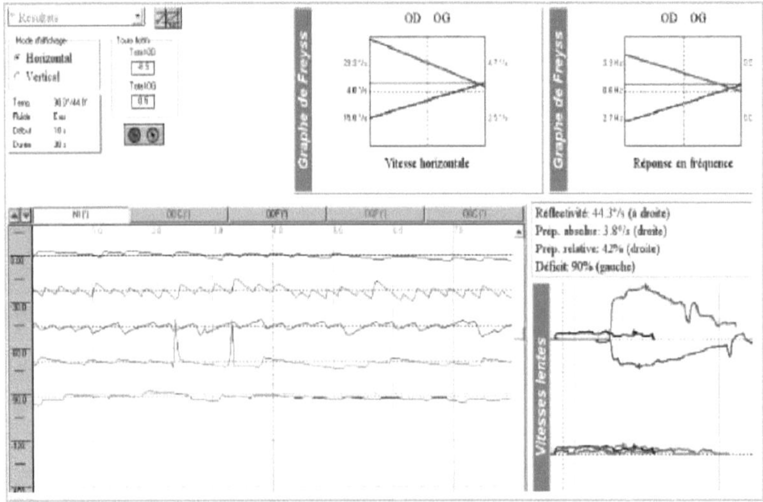

Figure 40: Left-hand side aerial view.

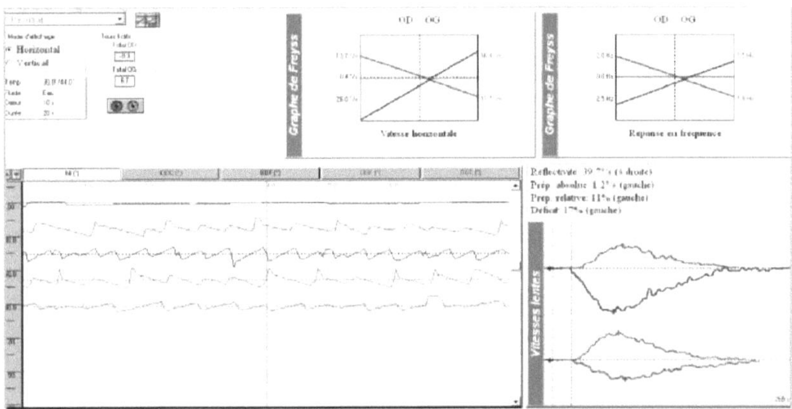

Figure 41: Compensated left hyporeflectivity.

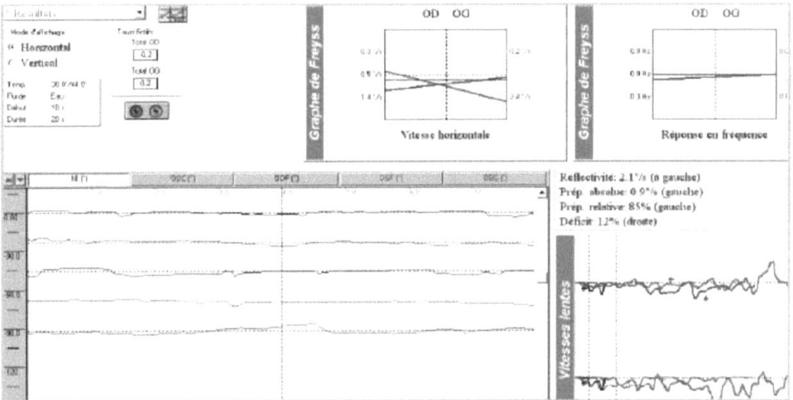

Figure 42: Uncompensated right hyporeflectivity.

SII-3-7: Visual Subjective Vertical (WS) and Visual Subjective Horizontal (HVS):

Perception of vertical and horizontal depends on otolith visual, proprioceptive and vestibular information.

In practice, the subject is placed in the dark in front of a luminescent cylindrical bar of 60 to 90 cm, oriented at 45°, and must turn it until it appears vertical.

If the mean deviation in VVS is less than 2.8° and 4° in HVS, the test is considered normal. Beyond that it becomes pathological and indicates either a peripheral otolith disorder, a central disorder or a visual disorder (astigmatism, oculomotor paralysis).

The VSL is not altered in bilateral vestibular damage. In the case of acute unilateral otolith injury, there is a significant deviation on the side of the injury. This deviation tends to disappear within a few weeks or months, due to vestibular compensation.

These tests cannot be used to determine whether the condition is peripheral or central.

SII-3-8: Video Head Impulse Test (VHIT):

This test consists of asking the subject to stare at a target located less than 1 m away while the examiner turns the head abruptly in the 6 planes of the canals. This test detects peripheral canal damage when the examiner makes a sudden movement of the head at a speed greater than 200° per second. At this speed, the optokinetic reflex is not involved in triggering the eye movement.

In the case of horizontal channel dysfunction, the gain of the vestibulo-ocular reflex is decreased and the subject cannot follow the instruction without making one or more refixation saccades to keep the eye on the target. These refixation saccades reflect high frequency channel dysfunction. This test allows the detection of overt saccades and the detection of covert saccades (Figures 42 and 43).

One of the great interests of the VHIT is that if it is normal in front of a neuritis picture, this is very suggestive of a central involvement and incites to ask for emergency imaging.

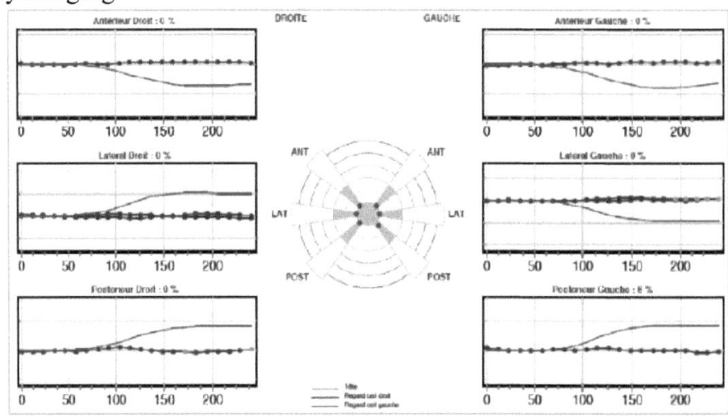

Figure 42: Representation of VHIT results in a normal subject

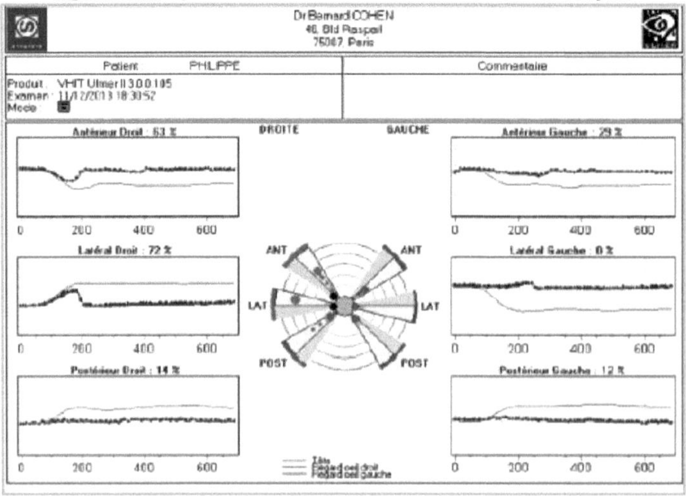

Figure 43: Representation of VHIT results in a subject with right lateral and anterior root canal dysfunction.

__III-3-9: Vibration test:__

This test allows the detection of a unilateral vestibular deficit (recent or old).

The method is simple: the head of the vibrator, whose frequency can be single, generally at 100Hz, or multiple, for example 30, 60, and 100Hz, is applied for 5 seconds on one mastoid, then on the other. The vibration stimulates all the sensors in the posterior labyrinth, on both the right and left sides, as the skull transmits the energy. Each sensor excited by the vibration responds but if they all have the same reactivity they cancel each other out. This test is of great value in cases of old vestibular lesions because the induced nystagmus often persists several years after the initial lesion.

Normal subjects do not have induced nystagmus. In case of asymmetry of function, a frank horizontal or horizonto-rotatory nystagmus is observed, greater than 3°/s, reproducible, non-exhaustible, beating on the healthy side whatever the stimulated side. It occurs without latency from the onset of stimulation and lasts for the duration of the stimulation. The nystagmus induced by the vibrator is clearly positive in peripheral vestibular disorders of the neuronitis type. However, it is sometimes present in the case of a central lesion, which does not allow us to confirm the peripheral origin of the damage when it is done in isolation.

__III-3-10: Otolithic evoked potentials (OEP):__

It was demonstrated in the 1950s that the saccule was activated by high intensity sound stimulation.

About 90% of the saccular PEO response comes from nerve fibres in the saccule, while 10% comes from the utricle and vice versa for the utricular PEO.

1/ Cervical evoked potentials :

The principle is as follows: sound clicks of 100dB are delivered unilaterally by means of a headset (air or bone stimulation) at a frequency of 5 Hz and myogenic potentials are collected bilaterally in the sternocleidomastoid muscles using surface electrodes placed in the upper third. Only the potentials collected in the muscle ipsilateral to the stimulation are of clinical interest.

During the recording, patients are placed in the supine position, raise their heads and turn them away from the sound stimulation so that the muscles are brought to maximum contraction.

Two early waves are collected P13 (negative) and N 23 (positive) after 10 and 19 ms respectively.

These early waves reflect the activation of paucisynaptic inhibitory sacculospinal pathways involving:

- a synapse between the saccular hair cells and the afferent endings of the saccular nerve;
- one or two synapses in the central vestibular nuclei;
- and finally a final synapse between the neuron endings

secondary vestibular and spinal motor neurons.

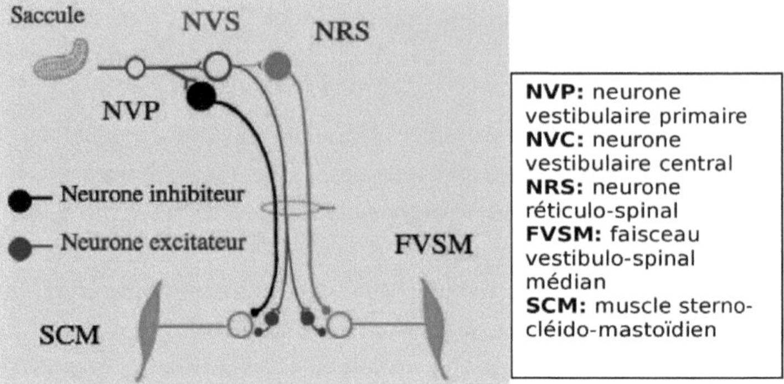

<u>Figure 44:</u> Neural pathways underlying myogenic evoked potentials

Two parameters are studied (Figure 45):

- Latency: it rarely varies in peripheral vestibular pathologies. On the other hand, it can be increased in the case of central pathology such as in multiple sclerosis.

- The amplitude of the P13/N23 peak: this depends on the amplitude of the electromyographic activity of the recorded SCM muscle and the type of stimulus administered. Therefore, it is of no value in the detection of a saccular lesion or sacculospinal pathways. For each stimulus, the ratio :

(amplitude on the healthy side - amplitude on the sick side)/

(amplitude on the healthy side + amplitude on the sick side).

An absence of early waves or a decrease in peak amplitude

P13/N23 on one side to the other by more than 50% indicates damage to the saccule and/or sacculospinal tract.

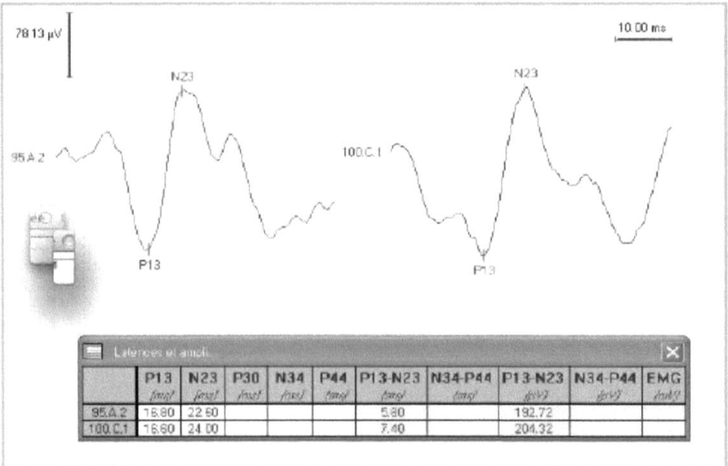

	P13	N23	P30	N34	P44	P13-N23	N34-P44	P13-N23	N34-P44	EMG
95.A.2	16.80	22.60				5.80		192.72		
100.C.1	16.60	24.00				7.40		204.32		

<u>Figure 45:</u> Representation of cervical otolith evoked potentials induced by high intensity sound stimuli.

42

This test is interesting when the symptomatology evoked by the patient is supposed to be otolithic: diplopia, floating, pitching sensations, tilting of the visual world. Moreover, it is not sensitive to compensation.

The diagnosis of endolymphatic fistula can be suspected when the PEO threshold is lowered below 85 dB.

Lack of response to PEO or prolonged latency of P13 and N23 waves suggests inferior vestibular nerve damage.

A potential limitation of this test is conductive hearing loss when the sound stimuli are delivered via the air. Indeed, the sound wave delivered at 100 dB does not reach the inner ear at an intensity sufficient to cause saccular activation. The P13 and N23 waves are therefore not found on the conductive side of the hearing loss, even though saccular function may be normal (false negative). However, the application of short tone bursts via the bone using a vibrator (500 Hz) allows the function of the saccular receptor to be assessed.

2/ Ocular evoked potentials (Figures 46):

The principle is as follows: the osseous or aerial stimulation of the otolith system is associated with the activation of the vestibulo-ocular reflex collected in the inferior oblique right eye muscle.

Two waves are collected n10 (positive) and p15 (negative).

PEOs collected under the right eye reflect the state of the left utricle and vice versa. Ocular OEPs that are absent, have long latencies or low amplitude (right/left asymmetry >35%) reflect dysfunction. Low frequency stimulation (250-500Hz) was better for Meniere's disease, while high frequency (1000-2000Hz) was better for superior canal dehiscence (increased amplitude of N10 on the side of the dehiscence). This test has a better sensitivity than the VVS in utricular pathology.

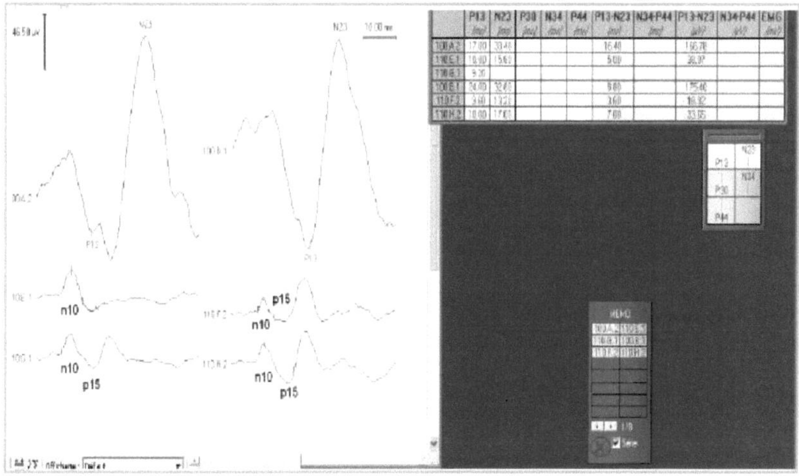

Figure 46: Representation of cervical and ocular otolithic evoked potentials induced by

sound stimuli.

The development of new techniques to explore vertigo has considerably facilitated its diagnostic and therapeutic approaches. Among these new techniques, videonystagmography (VNG) has a prominent place.

It allows the vestibular system to be studied in real time by observing the eye. The analysed data, associated with the clinical data, allow an etiological orientation in the case of any vertigo.

References

1 DE WAELE C. and TRAN BA HUY P.: Les vertiges et le praticien.

2 BONFILS C. AND PIERRE JM: ENT anatomy.

3 DEGUINE O. AND DARROUZET V: Electrophysiology in ENT, Société Française d'Oto- rhino-laryngologie et de Chirurgie de la Face et du Cou (2008).

4 GUINARD F.: Explorations vestibulaires. Encycl Méd Chir (Elsevier, Paris). Oto-rhino-laryngologie, 20-199-M-10, 1996, 23p.

5 ROMAN S, THORMASSIN JM: Vestibular physiology. EMC (Elsevier Paris), ORL 20- 198-A-10, 2000, 14p.

6 DE WAELE C, TRAN BA HUY P: Anatomy of the vestibular pathways. EMC (Elsevier paris) ORL 20-038-A-10. 2001.

7 M. TOUPET: Practical diagnosis of vertigo. EMC-Neurology 2. Elsevier (2005) 463474.

8 ERIK ULMER G: Videonystagmography in daily practice.

9: The courses of the DIU "vestibular rehabilitation" 2014-2015.

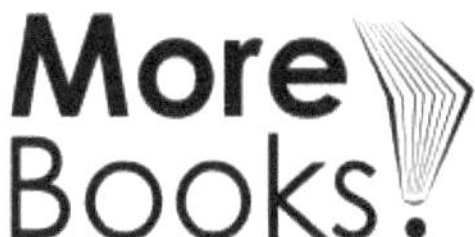

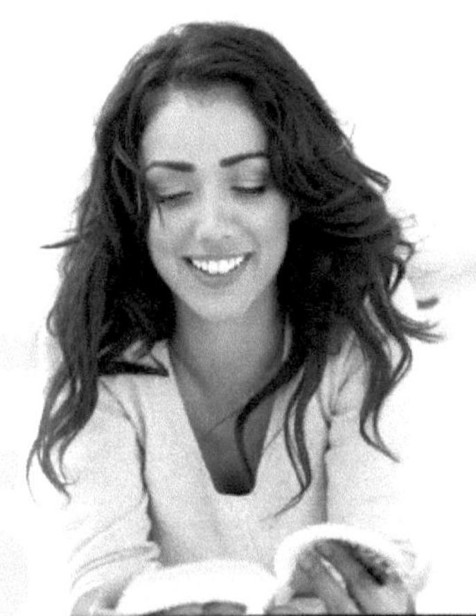

I want morebooks!

Buy your books fast and straightforward online - at one of world's fastest growing online book stores! Environmentally sound due to Print-on-Demand technologies.

Buy your books online at
www.morebooks.shop

Kaufen Sie Ihre Bücher schnell und unkompliziert online – auf einer der am schnellsten wachsenden Buchhandelsplattformen weltweit! Dank Print-On-Demand umwelt- und ressourcenschonend produziert.

Bücher schneller online kaufen
www.morebooks.shop

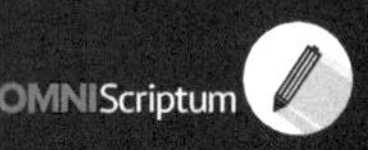

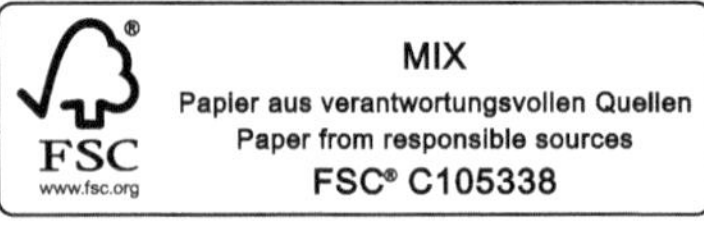

Printed by Books on Demand GmbH, Norderstedt / Germany